Simula SpringerBriefs on Computing

Volume 11

Springer and Simula have launched a new book series, *Simula SpringerBriefs on Computing*, which aims to provide introductions to select research in computing. The series presents both a state-of-the-art disciplinary overview and raises essential critical questions in the field. Published by SpringerOpen, all *Simula SpringerBriefs on Computing* are open access, allowing for faster sharing and wider dissemination of knowledge.

Simula Research Laboratory is a leading Norwegian research organization which specializes in computing. The book series will provide introductory volumes on the main topics within Simula's expertise, including communications technology, software engineering and scientific computing.

By publishing the *Simula SpringerBriefs on Computing*, Simula Research Laboratory acts on its mandate of emphasizing research education. Books in this series are published only by invitation from a member of the editorial board.

More information about this series at https://link.springer.com/bookseries/13548

Ahmed Elmokashfi • Olav Lysne • Valeriya Naumova

Editors

Smittestopp – A Case Study on Digital Contact Tracing

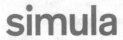

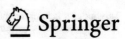

Editors
Ahmed Elmokashfi
SimulaMet
OsloMet – Oslo Metropolitan University
Oslo, Norway

Olav Lysne
SimulaMet
OsloMet – Oslo Metropolitan University
Oslo, Norway

Valeriya Naumova
Simula Consulting
Oslo, Norway

ISSN 2512-1677   ISSN 2512-1685 (electronic)
Simula SpringerBriefs on Computing
ISBN 978-3-031-05465-5   ISBN 978-3-031-05466-2 (eBook)
https://doi.org/10.1007/978-3-031-05466-2

Mathematics Subject Classification (2020): 92-XX, 94-XX

This Springer imprint is published by the registered company Springer Nature Switzerland AG
The registered company address is: Gewerbestrasse 11, 6330 Cham, Switzerland

Series Foreword

Dear reader,

Our aim with the series *Simula SpringerBriefs on Computing* is to provide compact introductions to selected fields of computing. Entering a new field of research can be quite demanding for graduate students, postdocs, and experienced researchers alike: the process often involves reading hundreds of papers, and the methods, results and notation styles used often vary considerably, which makes for a time-consuming and potentially frustrating experience. The briefs in this series are meant to ease the process by introducing and explaining important concepts and theories in a relatively narrow field, and by posing critical questions on the fundamentals of that field. A typical brief in this series should be around 100 pages and should be well suited as material for a research seminar in a well-defined and limited area of computing.

We have decided to publish all items in this series under the SpringerOpen framework, as this will allow authors to use the series to publish an initial version of their manuscript that could subsequently evolve into a full-scale book on a broader theme. Since the briefs are freely available online, the authors will not receive any direct income from the sales; however, remuneration is provided for every completed manuscript. Briefs are written on the basis of an invitation from a member of the editorial board. Suggestions for possible topics are most welcome and can be sent to mailto:aslak@simula.noaslak@simula.no.

January 2016

Prof. Aslak Tveito
CEO

Dr. Martin Peters
Executive Editor Mathematics
Springer Heidelberg, Germany

Preface

"Today, the Government launches the strongest and most intrusive restrictions ever imposed in Norway during peacetime."

Prime Minister Erna Solberg, 12 March 2020

A few hours after the prime minister's dramatic announcement, we addressed the Norwegian Institute of Public Health (NIPH) and offered our services. The day after, we were asked to develop a system based on mobile phones that could help trace the contacts of individuals infected by the coronavirus. The background of the request from NIPH was a very recent scientific paper subsequently published in the journal Science. [1] In short, it stated that, by using a reasonably efficient tracing system, the effect of the pandemic on society could be significantly reduced. The development of a system started the same evening and continued with 12- to 18-hour workdays for five weeks. The system was then launched by the prime minister and was quickly downloaded by about one-third of the population 16 years old and above. Privacy concerns and a major drop in infections resulted in halting the system about two months after it was launched.

This aim of this issue of the *Simula SpringerBriefs on Computing* is to describe in detail how the tracing system was built from a technical perspective. At the start of the project, time was of the essence and no one had ever built such a system. All technical issues within the project, therefore, had to be resolved, and as quickly as humanly possible. The present text describes these solutions. Our aim is to document what was done to be better prepared should a similar situation arise.

In Norway and in most parts of the Western world, contact tracing systems stirred up heated debate on privacy issues, and most countries ended up using systems based on a solution developed by Apple and Google. That system was strong in terms of privacy, but gave no information to the health authorities that could help support

---

[1] Ferretti, Luca, et al. "Quantifying SARS-CoV-2 transmission suggests epidemic control with digital contact tracing." Science 368.6491 (2020).

tracing the infection. In the end, these systems turned out to have very limited value from a public health perspective. The overall societal costs of applying a reduced system, in terms of deaths and lockdowns, are by now an open question. The decision to use the Apple/Google tool was enforced by Apple and Google through their control over the two main smartphone operating systems, leaving the health authorities little choice.[2] Whether such decisions should be made by technology companies or public health authorities is another open question.

By now, many contact tracing solutions have been developed, and it is our impression that, for these solutions, there is a constant trade-off between privacy and efficiency in the present state of knowledge. We can therefore develop systems of great efficiency and low privacy, or the other way around. Clearly, what we want is a system with great privacy and great efficiency, but, as far as we know, such a solution has not been developed or suggested in the growing literature on this topic. Our aim here is not to argue that our system (Smittestopp) achieved the right balance. It did not. Rather, our aim is to explain what we did and offer it to the scientific community so that others can improve both the efficiency and privacy of future solutions.

Oslo, Norway, September 2021,

Professor Aslak Tveito
CEO of Simula Research Laboratory

Professor Olav Lysne
Director of Simula Metropolitan
Center for Digital Engineering

Research Professor Ahmed Elmokashfi
Simula Metropolitan Center for
Digital Engineering

Dr. Valeriya Naumova
Director OF Simula Consulting

---

[2] Mark Scott, Elisa Braun, Janosch Delcker, and Vincent Manancourt, "How Google and Apple outflanked governments in the race to build coronavirus apps." Politico, May 2020, https://www.politico.eu/article/google-apple-coronavirus-app-privacy-uk-france-germany/.

Contents

4   Smittestopp analytics: Analysis of position data 63
Vajira Thambawita, Steven A. Hicks, Ewan Jaouen, Pål Halvorsen, and
Michael A. Riegler

5   Using Bluetooth for contact tracing 81
Ahmed Elmokashfi and Amund Kvalbein

Chapter 1
Introduction

Ahmed Elmokashfi, Olav Lysne, and Valeriya Naumova

1.1 Background

In the early months of 2020, a new virus began to spread in societies around the world. This virus, named SARS-CoV-2 or simply coronavirus, caused a disease called COVID-19 that had a deadly outcome in a disturbingly high fraction of cases. The elderly and those with an underlying chronic disease seemed to be particularly vulnerable [3]. Some months into 2020, the disease was classified as a global pandemic.

Diverse measures were taken in countries around the world to control the spread of the virus. These measures varied from nonintrusive advice on social distancing and hygiene to actual curfews where people were not allowed to leave their homes other than for strictly necessary errands.

Isolating infected individuals, identifying those with whom they have been in close contact, and asking them to isolate as well has emerged as a key strategy to break the chains of transmission of COVID-19. A process known as contact tracing is followed to identify close contacts. This process helped in slowing the SARS outbreak in early 2000 and is routinely used to break the transmission chains of sexually transmitted diseases. Conventional contact tracing is a largely manual process in which contact tracers interview infected individuals. It therefore scales

A. Elmokashfi
The Center for Resilient Networks and Applications, Simula Metropolitan Center for Digital Engineering,
e-mail: ahmed@simula.no

O. Lysne
The Center for Resilient Networks and Applications, Simula Metropolitan Center for Digital Engineering,
e-mail: Olav.lysne@simula.no

V. Naumova
Department of Machine Intelligence, Simula Metropolitan Center for Digital Engineering,
Simula Consulting AS, e-mail: valeriya@simula.no

poorly if the number of cases increases rapidly. It also misses unknown contacts, for example, encounters on public transportation.

One thing that distinguishes this pandemic from those of the past, however, is that most people, most of the time, are carrying powerful computing and communication devices in the form of mobile phones. These phones are expected to be equipped with Global Positioning System (GPS) functionality that could track their movements, Bluetooth functionality that could be leveraged to detect their proximity to other phones, and an Internet connection that could be used to transmit detection data to health authorities. Exploiting this already deployed technology to control the disease was therefore was an obvious path to explore.

In March 2020, a preprint of a research paper by recognized epidemiologists from the University of Oxford was circulated among health authorities in Europe. The paper's main conclusion was that, if the latency of tracing and quarantining the contacts of an infected person was reduced from days to hours, this by itself could suffice to stop the spread of the disease[4]. This reduction in latency is exactly what can be expected from introducing electronic contact tracing by the use of mobile phones.

From early March, development teams in many European countries tried to build an app-based contact tracing system. Their approaches varied, but the common denominator was that they all were attempting to use the Bluetooth technology that was deployed in phone models carried by most individuals, to detect when two people were physically sufficiently close to each other for a sufficiently long time for the transmission of the virus to take place.

Making Bluetooth work this way, however, was a nontrivial task. Bluetooth was not developed for this purpose and, at the outset there was no knowledge on the extent to which this would actually be possible, or how this would play out in the complex dynamics of human interaction and behaviour.

This book describes the Norwegian system for contact tracing that was developed in March and early April 2020. The system was deployed after five weeks of development and was active for a little more than two months, when a drop in infection levels in Norway and privacy concerns led to shutting it down.

The intention of this book is twofold. First, it reports on the design choices made in the development phase. Second, as one of the only systems in the world that collected population data into a central database and which was used for an entire population, we can share experience on how the design choices impacted the system's operation. By sharing lessons learned and the challenges faced during the development and deployment of the technology, we hope that this book can be a valuable guide for experts from different domains, such as big data collection and analysis, application development, and deployment in a national population, as well as digital tracing.

1.2 Timeline

When Norway closed down society on 12 March to stop the spread of COVID-19, several countries in Europe had already started to develop a contact tracing app. The Norwegian Institute of Public Health (NIPH) contacted Simula Research Laboratory and requested that we put aside other priorities and start the development of an app as quickly as possible. Given the severity of the situation, we agreed to do so. A development team was put together, and the development started on 13 March.

After initial considerations, the Norwegian authorities decided that the app should serve two purposes. The first purpose was to automate contact tracing, to start the quarantining of potentially infected people as efficiently and early as possible. The second purpose of the app was to collect information on Norwegian population's movements and interactions. This information was to be used at an aggregate level for the evaluation of shutdown measures implemented by the government to stop the pandemic. Aggregated and anonymized data was also to be kept for research purposes in preparation for future pandemics. A separate regulation for limiting the use of the collected data was passed in Parliament.

At the outset of this project, knowledge and research on the use of mobile phones for contact tracing was extremely scarce. A string of technical challenges therefore needed to be addressed. What the challenges were and how they were solved are discussed in the different chapters of this book.

The app we developed was named Smittestopp[1]. It was launched after a short and intense development phase that lasted five weeks, and, in the first few days after the launch, 1.5 million downloads of the app were registered. After two weeks of data collection, field tests of the system were started in three municipalities. At that time, however, the infection rate in Norway had dropped to almost zero. Field tests and validation of the system on real infected persons were therefore not possible.

The speed at which this system was developed must be considered in light of the sense of national crisis that reigned, both in the government and in the population at large. In a normal situation, such rapid development and deployment would be neither possible nor recommendable. A normal timeline for the development of such a product should be measured in months rather than weeks, and the time required by similar developments in other countries support this view.

On 10 April, Apple and Google announced that they were collaborating on creating an application programming interface (API) for contact tracing that would work seamlessly on both iOS and Android [2]. This was a very important development for several reasons. First, these two companies develop the two operating systems that are in use on almost all mobile phones in Norway. Integration of contact tracing into the operating system was therefore a very interesting prospect. Second, this new API promised efficient contact tracing without central data collection, and it therefore

---

[1] This term can be somewhat inaccurately translated as 'stop of infection'. Note that Smittestopp was later replaced by a GAEN based app that was also called Smittestopp. The two apps are not related.

appeared to have a far better privacy profile than any of the apps based on central storage that were being developed in Europe at the time.

The announcement from Apple and Google came six days before the planned launch of Smittestopp. Norwegian authorities still chose to launch the app as planned, for two reasons. The main reason was that a system based on the API from Apple and Google was at least two months away. In mid-April, the death rate due to infection was still high, and the main sentiment was there was no time to lose. The second reason was that the Norwegian authorities had decided that they needed data from the app to support their decision making regarding measures to shut down society. Google and Apple were very clear that any app based on their API could not send information to national authorities.

A few weeks after the launch of Smittestopp, the infection rate in Norway dropped to almost zero. The reduced need for the collection of data to control a pandemic, together with the advent of a more privacy-friendly technology in the form of Google and Apple's API, made the national authorities shut down Smittestopp after a little more than two months of operation.

At the time of this writing, most countries in Europe have terminated their own development of third-party contact tracing apps. The international community has converged on the use of Apple and Google's API. Still, in this book, we choose to tell the detailed story of the development of our third-party app. Our main reason for doing so is that we do not think that this is the last pandemic we will see. Furthermore, we do not think that the collaboration between Apple and Google is the final word with respect to digital contact tracing.

We firmly believe that, in the coming years, digital contact tracing should be an active research field, so that we are technologically better prepared next time. The outcome of such research will decide whether the mobile phone is a good platform for such tracing or if cheap and mass-produced specifically tailored hardware can be developed. Further outcomes of such research should be more accurate contract tracing algorithms and protocols with better privacy protection and that still give national authorities access to valuable anonymous information on how individuals, families, societies, and subcultures react to different pandemic control measures. We see this book as a major contribution to the literature on this topic.

1.3 Design choices

As discussed above, the design and development of the Smittestopp system took place in March and April 2020, immediately after the lockdown of Norwegian society. During the development phase, the Smittestopp team had to make a number of design choices to deliver the health authorities' requirements and handle the limitations that iOS imposes on the use of Bluetooth by apps running in the background, that is, apps that are launched and left running. The two key design choices were the use of centralized storage and the collection of GPS data.

The centralized storage of Bluetooth information offers a global view of contacts that helps in accommodating the inability of sleeping iPhones to detect neighbours. The Google/Apple Exposure Notifications (GAEN) API, which is now widely used by contact tracing apps, solves this problem in a decentralized manner. A recently published report containing a systematic comparison of a GAEN-based app and a Bluetooth-only Smittestopp app shows that, with centralized storage, Smittestopp can achieve the same level of utility as the GAEN-based app [1].

Despite the current consensus that contact tracing can be conducted on the basis of Bluetooth data alone, the second purpose of the intrinsic aggregation of descriptions of population mobility is to gain some level of access to the phones' locations over time, which necessitates the collection of GPS data. In addition, the health authorities wanted to leverage GPS data to contextualize contacts, to avoid false alarms that could lead to quarantining individuals that were not at any risk.

1.4 Team and project management

The project essentially consisted of two parallel projects, that is, one at NIPH [2] and one at Simula. NIPH's project focused on defining the requirements for harmonizing digital and manual contact tracing in an epidemiologically meaningful way, integrating with COVID testing databases, developing a system to inform app users who have been in close proximity to an infected individual, handling legal matters, as well as handling media and outreach. Simula's project focused mainly on developing the app, the backend needed for data storage, as well as developing the necessary analysis algorithms and tools. Several parties and companies were involved besides NIPH and Simula, including the Norwegian Directorate of eHealth, the Norwegian Health Network (NHN), and Microsoft. Furthermore, consultancy services were purchased from Scienta AS, Shortcut AS and Expert Analytics AS. Key people from NIPH and Simula met daily, including weekends, to discuss progress.

The project at Simula was split into three main teams:

1. *The app team*, which was responsible for developing and testing the app. This team comprised two sub-teams, for Android and iOS.
2. *The backend team*, which was responsible for designing and implementing the backend and implementing various APIs to facilitate communications between the phones and the backend. The task of designing the backend was a collaborative task, with contributions from NHN, Microsoft, and Simula. Microsoft helped by guiding Simula through Azure's capabilities, configuring the registration service, and implementing and managing the database. NHN was responsible for resource management and access control.
3. *The analytics team*, which had a set of broad responsibilities that included developing algorithms for estimating and contextualizing proximity and close contacts using GPS and Bluetooth, working closely with NIPH to tune and determine

---

[2] NIPH is called *Folkhelseinstituttet* in Norwegian.

how digital contact tracing could be used, developing systems for preparing and sharing contact tracing results with NIPH, and producing aggregate statistics at the national level.

In addition to these teams, two smaller teams provided communication and administrative support and coordinated security with NIPH. Overall, 22 Simula employees were involved in this effort. Each team had a number of daily meetings besides one general project meeting. All the development work was carried out at home during the lockdown period, where all meetings were virtual.

1.5 Smittestopp rollout

Smittestopp was launched on 16 April. The user registration service was overwhelmed on the day of the launch, which resulted in many users failing to complete their registration. In collaboration with Microsoft, a quick fix that significantly improved the system's scalability was deployed the next day. Between the launch and suspension dates, there were seven Smittstopp updates, three of them major releases. These updates enhanced various aspects, including power consumption, accessibility, and security. The most notable update was rolled out on 4 May, and it significantly improved the scanning of nearby Bluetooth devices on iOS.

Figure 1.1 plots the cumulative number of app downloads during Smittestopp's lifetime. The number of downloads climbed quickly, reaching 1.3 million on the second day after the launch. It then increased slowly to reach a maximum of 1.58 million on 2 June. The figure also shows that the number of downloads increased at

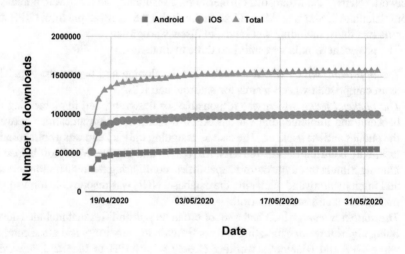

Fig. 1.1: The cumulative number of app downloads.

a much slower pace after the initial surge. This is expected, since there was no active campaign to encourage more users to download the app beyond the prime minister's appeal on the launch date.

Two-thirds of the downloads were by iOS devices. This was unexpected, given the state of the smartphone market in Norway. Through private communications with mobile network operators, we know that iPhones had a smartphone market share of about 55%, and Android phones had the rest. We cannot explain the difference without controlling for other factors, such as user age and location. Unfortunately, this could not be done, since Smittestopp has been halted indefinitely. However, understanding the causes of this difference could prove useful when releasing the next contact tracing application. Note that the cumulative downloads could include users who downloaded the app several times on the same phone. We do not know exactly the fraction of such downloads.

The total number of downloads gives an idea of the adoption of the app; however, the number of users who uploaded tracking data paints a better picture of the app's usage. Figure 1.2 depicts the number of unique users who uploaded data per day. This number was around 800,000 in the first three days, and then exhibited a decreasing trend, dropping to 450,000 by 4 June. Note that there is no one-to-one mapping between the largest number of daily users and the total number of users. Overall, about 1.2 million devices uploaded data during Smittestopp's lifetime. The number of unique users, however, could be slightly lower than 1.2 million, because some users might have completely reinstalled the app when updating to a new version. This would result in the same users having several identifiers and thus appearing as more than one user. We expect this fraction to be small, though. The gap between the number of downloads and the number of users, that is, approximately 300,000,

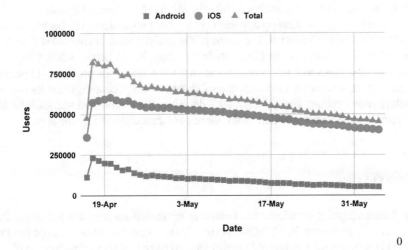

Fig. 1.2: Number of active users per day.

can have a number of reasons. First, a user might have updated the app several times, which translates into multiple downloads but not multiple users. Second, some users attempted to download the app several times on the launch date, due to the overloaded registration service. This translates to multiple downloads, but eventually only one of these downloads counting as a user. Finally, a fraction of users could have downloaded the app and removed it before it had uploaded any data. Bearing all these factors in mind, we believe that the number of users who downloaded and used Smittestopp was between 1 million and 1.2 million. In other words, between 23% and 27% of the Norwegian population older than 16 years downloaded and used Smittestopp. [3]

The loss of users was not uniform across the two platforms. One-third of iOS users were lost, compared to over two-thirds of Android users. We believe that this large difference can be blamed on the app resulting in higher battery consumption on Android. Optimizing the Android app proved difficult, due the great diversity in both vendors and devices. Accordingly, many users decided to uninstall the app to extend their battery life. In addition, many Android phones suspend apps that are not frequently used and consume large amounts of power, assuming that these apps are misbehaving and unnecessary.

These numbers show that Smittestopp was highly adopted in the beginning and continued to have a nontrivial level of adoption by the time it was shut down, that is, over 10% of the population. In the remainder of this book, we will go into more detail about Smittestopp and present its various components.

1.6 Book organization

The remainder of this book is divided into six standalone chapters. Chapter 2 provides an overview of the Smittestopp app for iOS and Android devices. The backend of the app is presented in Chapter 3. The scope of the analytic work is covered in Chapters 4 to 6. The processing of the GPS data is presented in Chapter 4, while Chapter 5 discusses how Bluetooth measurements are used to estimate the proximity of phones to each other. Chapter 6 discusses the validation of the technology and its use for digital contact tracing. Finally, Chapter 7 describes the mechanism and tools for the aggregation and anonymization of the movement data collected by the app.

References

[1] Sammenligning av alternative løsninger for digital smittesporing, Simula Research Laboratory, 2020, 2020. https://www.simula.no/sites/default/files/sammenligning_alternative_digital_smittesporing.pdf.

---

[3] The app was restricted to ages 16 and above.

[2] Apple and Google. Apple and google partner on covid-19 contact tracing technology. https://www.apple.com/newsroom/2020/04/apple-and-google-partner-on-covid-19-contact-tracing-technology/, Last visited July 2020, 2020.

[3] R.-H. Du, L.-R. Liang, C.-Q. Yang, W. Wang, T.-Z. Cao, M. Li, G.-Y. Guo, J. Du, C.-L. Zheng, Q. Zhu, et al. Predictors of mortality for patients with covid-19 pneumonia caused by sars-cov-2: a prospective cohort study. *European Respiratory Journal*, 55(5), 2020.

[4] L. Ferretti, C. Wymant, M. Kendall, L. Zhao, A. Nurtay, L. Abeler-Dörner, M. Parker, D. Bonsall, and C. Fraser. Quantifying SARS-CoV-2 transmission suggests epidemic control with digital contact tracing. *Science*, 368(6491), 2020.

Chapter 2
Smittestopp for Android and iOS

Per Magne Florvaag, Henrik Aasen Kjeldsberg, and Sebastian Kenji Mitusch

Abstract Contact tracing is currently a manual and laborious task that requires individuals to recall their interactions with people many days in the past. As a remedy, phones can be used to play a significant role in the response to the COVID-19 pandemic, by easing the burden of healthcare staff. Through novel and sophisticated technology, apps can be used to track infected people, issue quarantine guidelines, and provide the latest news to the public. Along with general public measures, apps can contribute significantly to keeping infection levels low. Generally, digital contract tracing can identify and warn people who may be at risk of being infected because they were in close physical proximity of someone who later tested positive for COVID-19.

2.1 Introduction

Our contact tracing app Smittestopp was released on 16 April 2020 on the Google Play store and Apple's App Store, and later for the Huawei AppGallery. The app supported Android 5.0+ and iOS 12.0+ and required users to register with a Norwegian phone number.

P.M. Florvaag
Department of Computational Physiology, Simula Research Laboratory,
Simula Consulting AS and Pacertool AS
e-mail: permagne@simula.no

H.A. Kjeldsberg
Department of Computational Physiology, Simula Research Laboratory,
e-mail: henriakj@simula.no

S.K. Mitusch
Department of Numerical Analysis and Scientific Computing, Simula Research Laboratory,
e-mail: sebastian@simula.no

© The Author(s) 2022
A. Elmokashfi et al. (eds.), *Smittestopp – A Case Study on Digital Contact Tracing*,
Simula SpringerBriefs on Computing 11, https://doi.org/10.1007/978-3-031-05466-2_2

To facilitate digital contact tracing, the apps had to collect information that could reveal the proximity between two devices running the app. If the devices are considered sufficiently close to each other, beyond a given threshold, and one (or both) of the users are later confirmed to be infected by COVID-19, the counterpart would be notified that they could be infected as well. The location data provided by Global Positioning System (GPS) can be used to match the locations of two users, but it is too coarse to distinguish distances to a precision of 2 metres, especially in cities and inside buildings. To counter this problem, Bluetooth data were supplied and combined with location data. Bluetooth signals fade rapidly over short distances, and one can semi-reliably determine distances with a precision of 2 metres.

GPS data are, however, very useful for the second purpose of the app: to gather anonymized movement patterns for epidemiological research. Specifically, the location data were intended to be used to evaluate the effect of social distancing measures imposed by the government.

For effective contact tracing, the app would need to run continuously in the background, even through phone reboots and app terminations. However, most users of such an app would open it once and then rarely or never open it again. As we will elaborate in this chapter, this proved to be a challenging aspect, especially for the iOS version of the app. More surprisingly, background location permissions would be essential for the life cycle of the app on iOS.

2.2 Related apps for digital contact tracing

Before the development of Smittestopp began, no digital contact tracing app had ever been released in a Western country. Although China had deployed apps to combat COVID-19, these apps functioned by showing the user's health status based on an algorithm that accounted for the user's travel history. Checkpoints were placed around China where a certain health status was required to pass through, such as when entering a metro station [28].

On 20 March 2020, Singapore released their digital contact tracing app TraceTogether [24]. TraceTogether gathers Bluetooth proximity data and stores them locally on the phone. The app fetches temporary identifiers from a central server and transmits these over Bluetooth. At the same time, the app builds a log of temporary identifiers it obtains from other devices in proximity. This contact log is then kept locally on the phone. When users tests positive for COVID-19, they can voluntarily share this contact log with the health authorities, who will then notify the other users. As other Bluetooth-based contact tracing apps on iOS, TraceTogether did not function properly in the background. Thus, iOS users were asked to use the app as a screen saver when not using the phone, ensuring that the app remained open and Bluetooth would work correctly [1].

On 22 March, Israel released their app HaMagen [23], which gathers location data through GPS (later versions also incorporate Bluetooth data). These data are stored locally on the phone until the user is diagnosed with COVID-19. Infected individuals can choose to upload these data so that other phones can download and compare these with their locally stored location history. The user is notified by the app if there is a match, but, to preserve privacy, the health authorities are not automatically notified.

The United Kingdom was initially developing a centralized contact tracing app using Bluetooth, but abandoned it in May, after reports that the background problems on iOS led to only a 4% detection rate between two iPhones that were asleep [18]. However, the importance of the 4% detection rate could have been overstated, since the quantity of contacts where both iPhones are asleep account for only a small percentage of overall contacts [19]. Instead, the UK government decided to switch to the Google/Apple Exposure Notifications (GAEN) application programming interface (API).

The GAEN API [26] is an API implemented by Google and Apple for both the Android and iOS operating systems. GAEN is similar to the *Decentralized Privacy-Preserving Proximity Tracing* (DP-3T) protocol [27], using only Bluetooth for proximity detection and storing all contact logs locally. However, a key difference between the two implementations is that the GAEN key matching occurs at the OS level, whereas that of the DP-3T protocol occurs at the app level. A GAEN app generates an identifier roughly every 15 minutes and transmits it over Bluetooth. When users test positive for COVID-19, they can choose to upload a log of the temporary keys they generated so that these can be downloaded by other users and matched against their locally stored contact logs. GAEN is currently the de facto standard framework for exposure notification.

2.3 App user interface and functionality

Smittestopp's user interface (UI) is mainly divided into four processes, or views. When the user starts Smittestopp for the first time, they are directed through the *onboarding* process. The onboarding process for both the Android and iOS apps is shown sequentially through the screenshots in Figure 2.1. The top row shows the process for Android, while the bottom one shows it for iOS. The onboarding is key to understanding Smittestopp, explaining the main purposes of the app, as shown in the first two panels (columns) of Figure 2.1. Furthermore, the onboarding presents the privacy policy, which the user is required to accept to continue using the app, shown in the third panel of Figure 2.1. Similarly, the user is required to verify that they are above the age of 16, a requirement for using Smittestopp, as shown in the fourth panel of Figure 2.1. In the iOS version, as shown in panel five of Figure 2.1, the onboarding page allows the user to authorize Smittestopp to collect Bluetooth and location service data. The user is given an authorization prompt in both versions of the app after login. Finally, the user is directed to the login services, provided by the Microsoft Authentication Library [22]. The login service requires users to input a Norwegian phone number and to authenticate themselves by replying with a confirmation code sent by SMS.

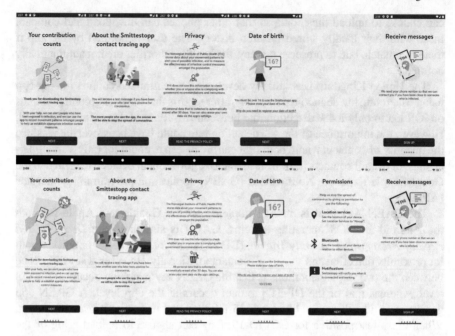

Fig. 2.1: Screenshots from Smittestopp's onboarding process. The top and bottom panels represent the onboarding flow in the Android and iOS versions of Smittestopp, respectively. Each flow involves up to six steps. Note that the Android version does not include the Permissions page.

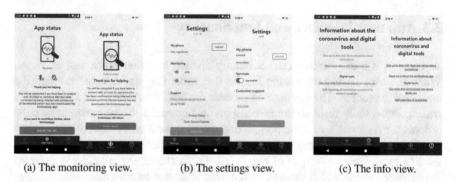

(a) The monitoring view.   (b) The settings view.   (c) The info view.

Fig. 2.2: The three view components after a successful login: monitoring, settings, and info. For all three images, the left and right screenshots represent the Android and iOS versions of Smittestopp, respectively.

After successfully logging in through Microsoft's service, the user is presented with the *monitoring* page, as shown in Figure 2.2a. The monitoring page serves as an overview of the app's status, which is either **enabled**, **partly enabled**, or **disabled**, although the wording can vary between apps. In Figure 2.2a, the app is fully enabled, implying the collection of both Bluetooth and location service data has been authorized and is activated.

In contrast, when partly enabled, that is, when either Bluetooth or location services are disabled, a button prompting the user to toggle the respective setting is shown. However, the collection of either data type will still contribute to the app's purposes, although the precision could be affected. Finally, if the monitoring shows the disabled status, then both Bluetooth and location services have been deactivated, either through the app's settings or through the phone's settings.

The supplementary view components consist of the settings and info views, shown in Figures 2.2b and 2.2c, respectively. The settings page displays the phone number with which the app was registered and the ability to log out, which temporarily halts the data collection. The user can also toggle the information that is collected. Customer support information is presented in the next settings panel, including a link to Helsenorge.no and its support phone number. In this panel, the user can also erase all the data collected by Smittestopp thus far. Finally, the *Info* view, shown in Figure 2.2c, displays helpful links related to Smittestopp, data collection, and general information about COVID-19.

2.4 System architecture and data flow

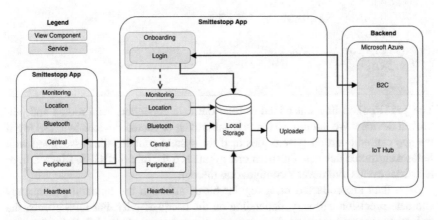

Fig. 2.3: High-level schematic of Smittestopp showing the main components and how they interact with the backend, through Microsoft services here, and with other devices where Smittestopp is installed. The backend consists of Azure Active Directory Business-to-Consumer (Azure AD B2C) and the Azure Internet of Things (IoT) Hub, which connects to the cloud.

A software architecture establishes the fundamental structure of a software system and displays how a collection of components accomplishes a specific task or function.

The main functions of Smittestopp are to aggregate location and Bluetooth data, with minor functions, such as the logging of events and heartbeat monitoring. The main components are presented in Figure 2.3, which is a high-level schematic overview of the process flow in Smittestopp. Although there are minor technical differences between the Android and iOS apps, the main components and data processing in Smittestopp are covered by the schematic.

Starting with their onboarding, users proceed through a login service provided by Azure AD B2C. The users input their Norwegian phone number and receive an access token from Azure AD B2C that is used to authenticate the user for Azure IoT Hub. The IoT hub responds with an authentication key and a Universally Unique Identifier (UUID), which are stored locally on the user's device. The authentication key is used to generate temporary authentication tokens for sending messages to the IoT hub. These messages are sent over HTTPS, with a payload as described below, in addition to the device's UUID.

After successfully logging in, the user is presented with the monitoring view component. Here, three main data types are actively collected and uploaded to the IoT hub, assuming full authorization to location services (GPS) and Bluetooth Low Evergy (BLE). All three events include five common fields, along with the event data, as shown in the following JavaScript Object Notation (JSON) message format example.

```
{
    "appVersion": "1.1.0",
    "model": " iPhone 10,5",
    "events": [EventData],
    "platform": "ios",
    "osVersion": "13.4.1",
    "jailbroken": false
}
```

The `jailbroken` flag was added to filter out data collection from rooted and jailbroken devices. We attempt to identify jailbroken or rooted devices by checking if the app can edit certain system files or if the system contains files associated with jailbroken/rooted devices. Furthermore, events is a list of either GPS, Bluetooth, or heartbeat events, but never a combination thereof.

GPS data are collected on a regular basis, although the uploading frequency and data precision can vary, depending on the user's activity. For GPS events, the following example message format shows the structure of the IoT hub telemetry message sent from the app to the cloud, including the common fields addressed above.

```
{
    "timeFrom": "2020-04-30T12:38:30Z",
    "timeTo": "2020-04-30T12:38:30Z",
    "latitude": 61.93372532454498,
    "longitude": 10.728583389659596,
```

```
  "accuracy": 65.0,
  "speed": 2.10,
  "altitude": 71.1960678100586,
  "altitudeAccuracy": 10.0
}
```

Newly collected GPS data are aggregated with previous GPS events for the period lasting from `timeFrom` to `timeTo`. The current location is determined by the `latitude` and `longitude` coordinates, along with the `altitude` above sea level, measured in metres. The `accuracy` and the `altitudeAccuracy` are measures of the location and altitude accuracy, respectively. In addition, the measured `speed` of the device, in metres per second, is registered [14, 8].

Devices that support BLE, particularly Android and iOS devices, can act as a peripheral device and a central device, as explained further in Section 2.6.3. As illustrated in Figure 2.3, a device acting as a central device can be detected by peripheral devices, which triggers an exchange of UUIDs between the devices involved. In the initial release of Smittestopp, devices used static UUIDs. However, the use of static UUIDs can expose user devices to tracking by scanners configured to detect Smittestopp UUIDs. As a remedy, rotating UUIDs can be used, an improvement that was later implemented and tested but never released to the public, because Smittestopp was abruptly halted. To link the BLE information to GPS data, the BLE data are aggregated with the last known GPS positions, saved in the `location` field, as shown in the following message format representing a BLE event.

```
{
  "deviceId": "123456789 abcd",
  "rssi": -90,
  "txPower": 12,
  "time": "2020-04-30T12:38:30Z",
  "location": {
    "latitude": 61.93372532454498,
    "longitude": 10.728583389659596,
    "accuracy": 65.0,
    "timestamp": "2020-04-30T12:35:30Z"
  }
}
```

The contact timestamp is registered in the `time` field, along with the UUID, `deviceId`, of the discovered device. Here, `rssi` represents the signal strength that the central device receives, while `txPower` represents the transmission power of the peripheral device.

The third and final event consists of heartbeat messages, a custom message used to determine a device's authorization of location services. The heartbeat message can also determine that the app is still installed and running on a device. A heartbeat event is sent once every 24 hours to the IoT hub, and it includes information on which

kind of data collection is enabled on the device, as shown in the following message
format.

```
{
  "timestamp": "2020-04-30T12:38:30Z",
  "state": 0
}
```

Here, the timestamp is updated when the message is uploaded, and the integer value
of state is set to one of four values.

Smittestopp is also connected to Azure App Center for logging purposes [20].
Note that the App Center is used by the app in parallel to the main app services,
thus running independently of the Smittestopp backend. Mainly errors and warnings
are logged and uploaded to the App Center, including information about failed
authorization, database errors, and failed requests and responses related to event
uploading. In addition, the operating system, mobile operator, version number, and
phone model is added to the App Center payload, used to improve the quality of
the collected data by distinguishing different phone models and operating systems.
Azure App Center does not store any personal information or link the collected data
to a user [21]. It is important to emphasize that the information collected by App
Center was only used to identify problems with certain phone models or operating
systems.

2.5 App life cycle

Whether running on the iOS or Android operating system, every mobile app passes
through multiple states throughout its runtime, known as the app's life cycle. Of the
different states an app can transition through, we mainly focus on those when the app
is running in the background, since most users of Smittestopp rarely opened the app.
Users bring apps to the foreground to interact with them. Consequently, such apps
will be prioritized when it comes to accessing systems resources. In contrast, apps in
the background are not visible to users. An app goes into the background if has been
stopped or has entered a suspended state. Most apps are usually in a background or
suspended state, to save as much power as possible. Optimally, the app does as little
work as possible, preferably nothing when off-screen. There are also intermediate
states, when the app's state changes from the foreground to the background and vice
versa, but these are not our focus here.

2.5.1 Android

Smittestopp supports Android 5.0+ and controls its life cycle through different
activities, as shown in Figure 2.4. The different activities describe the actions that

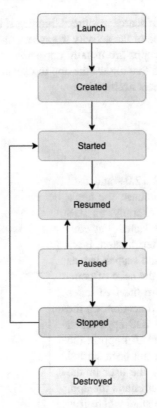

Fig. 2.4: A state diagram that describes the transitions between the states for the Android life cycle.

users can perform to make the app enter different life cycle states. An Android app cycles between the four following life cycle states: active, paused, stopped, and terminated [16]. The states are entered through different activities, which we describe next.

The app becomes active by going through the three activities *create*, *start*, and *resume*. When the user opens an app, the create activity is triggered. The app continues by executing the start activity. In this phase, the activity is still not rendered, but is about to become visible to the user. The final phase of being active involves the app entering the resume activity, where the app is finally visible to the user and becomes interactive.

At this point the app can be paused, stopped, or terminated. In the paused state, the app can still be visible to the user, but the user cannot interact with it. This state can be entered when the app is no longer in focus or before transitioning to the stopped or terminated state. The app enters the stopped state when it is not visible to the user, which can happen if a new activity is started or the current one is being terminated. Although the app is still active in the background, Android Runtime can terminate the app in case of scarce resources. Finally, if the app is terminated, it will destroy the current instance of the activity to save memory.

Considering that most apps are usually not active, we used a designated background service in Android that allows the app to execute events in the background, as well as showing a constant notification.

2.5.2 iOS

Smittestopp supports iOS 12.0+ and uses app delegate objects to manage the app's shared behaviours [9]. Generally, an iOS app can enter one of five states that constitute the app life cycle: terminated, inactive, active, background, and suspended, as shown in Figure 2.5. For the sake of completeness, we describe here the five states before focusing, in the next section, on the main challenges faced by iOS apps when they run in the background. An app in the *terminated* state has either not been started yet or has been closed by the user or the system. As soon as the user enters the app, the enters an intermediate state where it is *inactive*. In the inactive state, the app's UI is not visible to the user and does not receive or send any events. The inactive state is also entered every time the app transitions to a different state.

When the app is fully loaded, the app enters the *active* state. In the active state, the app is fully functional and visible to the

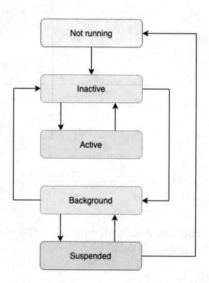

Fig. 2.5: A state diagram describing the transitions between the states for the iOS life cycle.

user and the user can interact with the UI. Additionally, the app can both send and receive events if this is part of the its functionality. When the user exits the app, it transitions from the active state to the inactive state before reaching the *background* state. Similarly, when reopening, the app will transition from the background state to the inactive state before eventually becoming active. The background state is usually only a temporary state in which the app's code is still executed, meaning that events can be sent and the app works in the background, although the UI is not visible to the user. After being in the background state for a short time, the app will enter the *suspended* state. The time it takes before the app transitions from the background state to the suspended state can vary, since this state can be extended, if needed, by the app. Most apps are automatically suspended by the system after entering the background state. In this state, the app does not execute code, but it is still saved in the iPhone's memory without affecting the battery life. In case the system runs low on memory, a suspended app can automatically be terminated by the system. An app can also enter the terminated state if it is manually terminated by the user.

2.6 Design choices

In this section, we discuss the various design choices that we made when developing the Smittestopp app. Section 2.6.1 gives a short description of how data are stored locally on the device and the security measures implemented for this storage. Battery usage is a prominent issue for a continuously running app such as Smittestopp, especially considering that it provides no immediate and obvious benefit to the user. Most of the battery drain was caused by location tracking, and details on how this was handled are provided in Section 2.6.2.Finally, Section 2.6.3 describes how proximity detection over Bluetooth was implemented.

2.6.1 Storage and security

Local storage consists of two different systems. One system is for preference data, such as the phone number, consent to the privacy policy, and the login token. The other system is a local encrypted SQLite database for measurement data, such as location and Bluetooth encounters. Preference data are stored in UserDefaults and the Keychain [7] on iOS, and in SharedPreferences and Keystore [13] on Android. Keychain and Keystore are used to store sensitive information such as the phone number, the login token, and the encryption key for the local SQLite database.

The local database system choice was SQLite [25] because it is an embedded database with easily accessible libraries. On Android, SQLite is part of the AndroidX library [15]. On iOS, an open source library was used [12]. The database consists of two tables, one for GPS data and one for BLE data. As the data are being uploaded, they are marked for deletion and, upon successful upload, the marked data are deleted. Since the location and proximity data can persist on a phone for hours before they are successfully uploaded, it is important that they are stored as securely as possible. This entails the entire database being encrypted using a key that is generated and stored on the device in Keychain (iOS) or Keystore (Android). Although someone with full access to the phone could theoretically access the encryption key, this database encryption provides a basic level of security.

2.6.2 Location services

The collection of location data in Smittestopp is performed for two purposes: for digital contact tracing in combination with BLE event data and for gathering movement patterns in the population for epidemiological research, to understand the effectiveness of recommended public measures. By default, both the Android and iOS apps fetch location data at regular intervals, merging similar location data points to avoid sending too much data. However, the continuous tracking of location services was one of the main power usages of Smittestopp, as reflected in the number of reviews on both Apple's App Store and the Google Play store complaining about the app's impact on battery life.To address the high power consumption, Smittestopp would change the accuracy of the GPS data adaptively.

While, on Android, only the intervals at which location data were retrieved was tweaked, the iOS version of Smittestopp combined multiple different features of the CoreLocation [2] framework. By default, the app uses the standard `CoreLocation` location updates with the highest possible precision. If the GPS data show the same position, or roughly the same within a threshold dependent on the GPS accuracy, for more than five minutes, high precision location updates are disabled and, instead, *region monitoring* [10] is used. Region monitoring, also known as geofencing, constructs a circular region around a position with a given radius and tracks if the user moves outside the region. The region is defined as a circle with a 40-metre radius around the last known position. iOS then alerts the app once the device moves outside the region and stays outside for at least 20 seconds.

When an iOS user grants Smittestopp permission to fetch location data in the background, the iOS app can run continuously in the background state, never moving to suspended state. The standard location updates [4] in the `CoreLocation` framework prevent the app from being suspended when moving to the background. However, turning off standard location updates would mean the app will be suspended. Thus, when switching to region monitoring, standard location updates are not turned off, but the accuracy is significantly lowered and the filter for how far apart each update needs to be is significantly increased. This means the app remains enabled but there will be no standard location updates, which prevents the app from moving to the suspended state.

Apart from the suspended state, the terminated state could also be a problem for Smittestopp on iOS. The app could enter the terminated state if the user manually terminated the app, which, one can imagine, is a very normal occurrence; however, when the user moves outside the currently monitored region, the app is launched automatically by the operating system [5]. In addition, a `CoreLocation` feature called *significant location updates* [4], which provides updates if the device moves by roughly 500 metres or more, is always enabled. Region monitoring and significant location updates in conjunction meant that, after app termination, the app would relaunch and continue as normal if the device moved 40 to 500 metres from its last known position.

Although the app could run continuously in the background, on iOS, this was entirely dependent on the user granting full background location permissions. Without those permissions, the app would not be able to gather location data in the background and would almost entirely rely on Bluetooth to wake the app. Because the Bluetooth background mode does not work after app termination and most users will not regularly launch the app, the iOS version of Smittestopp was extremely reliant on full location permissions for long-term consistency. This point was made tougher by iOS 13, which does not allow for background location permissions to be asked directly. Instead, one can only ask for permissions when the app is in use, and the user would later, at the discretion of the operating system, be prompted for background location permissions. This made it difficult to communicate to users what permissions they should grant, and the released version of Smittestopp did not attempt to convey the importance of background location permissions.

2.6.3 Bluetooth Low Energy

Bluetooth Low Energy (BLE) communication consists of two devices: one device advertising its presence and the other scanning for advertising BLE devices. BLE advertisement packets usually contain one or more UUIDs that inform the scanning devices of the types of services supported by the device in question. Such a UUID is referred to as a service UUID. The Smittestopp app advertises and scans for a service UUID specific to the app, providing a way for the scanning device to detect devices in its proximity. While BLE supports attaching some (limited size) data to the advertisement packet, there is limited support for accessing these data on iOS devices. Specifically, the data are not accessible when the scanning device has Smittestopp running in the background, and not in the foreground. Thus, Smittestopp instead connects to the advertising device when the app-specific service UUID is present. These connections are short-lived, since the scanning device only requests a device identifier from the advertising device and disconnects as soon as this has been received.

Running BLE in the background on an iOS app is supported through background modes, but the app will be suspended after a few seconds in the background. It will then transition from the suspended to the background mode every time a relevant BLE service UUID is found in a received advertisement packet or when a device connects. The app will then have approximately 30 seconds in the background state before it is suspended again.

Additionally, when the iOS app is in the background, the advertisement packet for the app changes to a proprietary format in which service UUIDs are found in the so-called overflow area [11]. The overflow area is a 128-bit array, and each service UUID corresponds to exactly one of the bits being set to one. When an iOS device scans for a specific service UUID, it will match advertisements where the corresponding bit is set to one. Of course, service UUIDs can be 128-bit numbers, for a many-to-one mapping from a service UUID. Thus, there is a possibility that a false positive can be detected if a device advertises a service UUID that has the same corresponding overflow area bit. For more information on the overflow area, see the notes by Rossum [29] and Young [30].

While the BLE stack in iOS has a built-in system for handling the overflow advertisement format, an Android device does not know how to translate service UUIDs to their corresponding bit. To do so, the Android implementation of Smittestopp, in addition to scanning for the normal app-specific service UUID, also scans for packets with the corresponding bit set to one. Since the code for mapping service UUIDs to a bit is not public, the bit is found by scanning the BLE advertisement packets that the iOS app transmits in the background. This is possible because the corresponding bit is always the same for a specific service UUID.

The difficulties with BLE on iOS while the app is in the background are not only limited to the advertisement packets. When the scanning app is in the background, iOS will not relay any overflow advertisement packets detected to the app. Thus, while in the background state, an iOS app will not be able to detect other backgrounded iOS apps. While the app will function fine between iOS and Android devices, detection between two backgrounded iOS apps will not work. Furthermore, more than half of the phone users in Norway use an iPhone. Because the average user will have the app almost exclusively in the background state, this was a major problem and one of the main topics in meetings with collaborating countries.

In early April, two weeks before the app would eventually launch, we discovered a way to partially circumvent this limitation. Using the iBeacon feature [6], found in the CoreLocation [2] framework, the operating system will continue to relay overflow advertisement packets to the app, even in the background. Specifically, by ranging for iBeacons [3], a method that allows one to determine the proximity of other devices with iBeacon, the app can continue to receive overflow advertisements while the device screen is on. The iBeacons for which the app scans do not have to be present at all. The app can scan for a random iBeacon UUID. However, if the device screen is off, this method will not help the app detect BLE advertisements. Notably, whether the device is locked or not does not matter, as long as the screen is on. This means that if, for example, the phone is locked but receives a notification, it will light up and the app will receive BLE advertisements until the screen goes black again. With this workaround, it is possible to detect all encounters where at least one phone is in use. This method is also briefly mentioned by Young [30].

Although ranging for an iBeacon would help with BLE detection, a major concern was the impact on battery life. Hence, we aimed to minimize the time the app spends ranging for an iBeacon. The documented iOS app API from Apple does not include a way to detect whether the phone screen is on or off. Therefore, the app potentially ranges for an iBeacon when it has no effect, negatively impacting the battery life for no benefit. However, using an undocumented API, we can register callbacks that are invoked when the screen is turned off or on. The use of such undocumented APIs usually means that the app will be rejected in the App Store review process, and Apple made no exception for Smittestopp regarding this matter. Thus, the Smittestopp app ended up ranging for an iBeacon every five minutes for 10 seconds, regardless of whether the screen is on or off.

Ranging for iBeacons requires location permissions on iOS, even when only used to improve BLE background consistency. Additionally, to turn iBeacons on and off while in the background, the app must not be in a suspended state and must have background location permissions. From the user's perspective, requiring location permissions to improve BLE capabilities is not intuitive. Communicating the need for location permissions is therefore a significant challenge for an app using this workaround.

2.7 Testing

Smittestopp's codebase was tested using unit tests for the functionality, UI, and snapshot tests [17] to test the UI. The UI tests simulate interactions with the UI and check for the expected behaviour. Meanwhile, Snapshot tests compare old screenshots of the UI to the current UI, to ensure that no unintended changes occur.

2.8 Conclusions and lessons learned

Designing an app that runs almost exclusively in the background is much more straightforward on Android than on iOS. To conserve battery life, most iOS apps are not allowed to execute code when they are backgrounded, and, even if an app asks for time in the background, the iOS system will only rarely or even never grant background execution time if the app is rarely used.

Furthermore, the iOS system limits the functionality of BLE in the background. This limitation can be partially alleviated by background location permissions, but the user must explicitly grant these. This is perhaps a good thing from a privacy perspective, since it makes it difficult for apps to implement tracking mechanisms over BLE. However, it was one of the main challenges for countries implementing BLE contact tracing apps.

References

[1] G. T. Agency. 6 things about OpenTrace, the open-source code published by the TraceTogether team. `https://www.tech.gov.sg/media/technews/six-things-about-opentrace\#6-last-but-not-least-an-extra-step-for-ios-users`, 2020 (accessed October 26, 2020).

[2] Apple Developer Documentation. Core Location. `https://developer.apple.com/documentation/corelocation/`, 2020 (accessed October 26, 2020).

[3] Apple Developer Documentation. Determining the Proximity to an iBeacon Device. `https://developer.apple.com/documentation/corelocation/determining_the_proximity_to_an_ibeacon_device`, 2020 (accessed October 26, 2020).

[4] Apple Developer Documentation. Getting the User's Location. `https://developer.apple.com/documentation/corelocation/getting_the_user_s_location`, 2020 (accessed October 26, 2020).

[5] Apple Developer Documentation. Handling Location Events in the Background. `https://developer.apple.com/documentation/corelocation/getting\_the\_user\_s\_location/handling_location_events_in_the_background`, 2020 (accessed October 26, 2020).

[6] Apple Developer Documentation. iBeacon. `https://developer.apple.com/ibeacon/`, 2020 (accessed October 26, 2020).

[7] Apple Developer Documentation. Keychain Services. `https://developer.apple.com/documentation/security/keychain_services`, 2020 (accessed October 26, 2020).

[8] Apple Developer Documentation. Location Services. `https://developer.apple.com/documentation/corelocation/cllocationmanager`, 2020 (accessed October 26, 2020).

[9] Apple Developer Documentation. Managing Your App's Life Cycle. `https://developer.apple.com/documentation/uikit/app_and_environment/managing_your_app_s_life_cycle`, 2020 (accessed October 26, 2020).

[10] Apple Developer Documentation. Monitoring the User's Proximity to Geographic Regions. `https://developer.apple.com/documentation/corelocation/monitoring_the_user_s_proximity_to_geographic_regions`, 2020 (accessed October 26, 2020).

[11] Apple Developer Documentation. startAdvertising(_:). `https://developer.apple.com/documentation/corebluetooth/cbperipheralmanager/1393252-startadvertising`, 2020 (accessed October 26, 2020).

[12] S. Celis. A type-safe, Swift-language layer over SQLite3. `https://github.com/stephencelis/SQLite.swift`, 2020 (accessed October 26, 2020).

[13] A. Developers. Android keystore system. `https://developer.android.com/training/articles/keystore`, 2020 (accessed October 26, 2020).

[14] A. Developers. Android location services. `https://developer.android.com/reference/android/location/Location`, 2020 (accessed October 26, 2020).

[15] A. Developers. Sqlite. `https://developer.android.com/jetpack/androidx/releases/sqlite`, 2020 (accessed October 26, 2020).

[16] A. Developers. Understand the Activity Lifecycle. `https://developer.android.com/guide/components/activities/activity-lifecycle`, 2020 (accessed October 26, 2020).

[17] Github.   Delightful Swift snapshot testing.   `https://github.com/pointfreeco/swift-snapshot-testing`, 2020 (accessed October 23, 2020).

[18] L. Kelion. Coronavirus: England's contact-tracing app gets green light for trial. `https://www.bbc.com/news/technology-53753678`, 2020 (accessed October 23, 2020).

[19] L. Kelion. Coronavirus: Ireland set to launch contact-trace app. `https://www.bbc.com/news/technology-53137816`, 2021 (accessed February 18, 2021).

[20] Microsoft Azure. Visual Studio App Center. `https://azure.microsoft.com/en-us/services/app-center`, 2020 (accessed October 26, 2020).

[21] Microsoft Azure. Visual Studio App Center. `https://docs.microsoft.com/en-us/appcenter/gdpr/faq\#data-use`, 2021 (accessed February 25, 2021).

[22] Microsoft Azure. Microsoft Authentication Library (MSAL). `https://docs.microsoft.com/en-us/azure/active-directory/develop/msal-overview`, 2021 (accessed February 26, 2021).

[23] I. M. of Health. HaMagen. `https://govextra.gov.il/ministry-of-health/hamagen-app/download-en/`, 2020 (accessed October 23, 2020).

[24] G. of Singapore. TraceTogether. `https://www.tracetogether.gov.sg/`, 2020 (accessed October 26, 2020).

[25] SQLite. SQLite Home Page. `https://www.sqlite.org/`, 2020 (accessed October 26, 2020).

[26] P.-P. C. Tracing. Apple and Google. `https://covid19.apple.com/contacttracing`, 2020 (accessed October 26, 2020).

[27] C. Troncoso, M. Payer, J.-P. Hubaux, M. Salathé, J. Larus, E. Bugnion, W. Lueks, T. Stadler, A. Pyrgelis, D. Antonioli, et al. Decentralized privacy-preserving proximity tracing. *arXiv preprint arXiv:2005.12273*, 2020.

[28] J. Utzerath, R. Bird, and G. Cheng. Contact tracing apps in China, Hong Kong, Singapore and South Korea. `https://www.lexology.com/library/detail.aspx?g=99dca469-455d-4f7a-b025-00bf1d10ff6b`, 2020 (accessed October 23, 2020).

[29] A. van Rossum. Smartphone localization. `https://github.com/crownstone/bluenet-ios-basic-localization/blob/master/BROADCASTING_AS_BEACON.md`, 2020 (accessed October 26, 2020).

[30] D. G. Young. Hacking The Overflow Area. `http://www.davidgyoungtech.com/2020/05/07/hacking-the-overflow-area`, 2020 (accessed October 26, 2020).

Chapter 3
Smittestopp Backend

Cise Midoglu, Benjamin Ragan-Kelley, Sven-Arne Reinemo, Jon Jahren and Pål Halvorsen

Abstract An efficient backend solution is of great importance for any large-scale system, and Smittestopp is no exception. The Smittestopp backend comprises various components for user and device registration, mobile app data ingestion, database and cloud operations, and web interface support. This chapter describes our journey from a vague idea to a deployed system. We provide an overview of the system internals and design iterations and discuss the challenges that we faced during the development process, along with the lessons learned. The Smittestopp backend handled around 1.5 million registered devices and provided various insights and analyses before being discontinued a few months after its launch.

C. Midoglu
Department of Holistic Systems, Simula Metropolitan Center for Digital Engineering,
e-mail: cise@simula.no

B. Ragan-Kelley
Department of Numerical Analysis and Scientific Computing, Simula
e-mail: benjaminrk@simula.no

S.A. Reinemo
Simula Metropolitan Center for Digital Engineering,
e-mail: svenar@simula.no

J. Jahren
Microsoft, Norway,
e-mail: Jon.Jahren@microsoft.com

P. Halvorsen
Department of Holistic Systems, Simula Metropolitan Center for Digital Engineering,
Department of Computer Science, Oslo Metropolitan University,
Department of Informatics, University of Oslo
e-mail: paalh@simula.no

A. Elmokashfi et al. (eds.), *Smittestopp − A Case Study on Digital Contact Tracing*,
Simula SpringerBriefs on Computing 11, https://doi.org/10.1007/978-3-031-05466-2_3

3.1 Introduction

The COVID-19 pandemic struck Europe very hard in the spring of 2020. In Norway, manual tracing was successfully used to identify and quarantine close contacts of confirmed cases to some extent, helping reduce the spread of the disease. However, since manual tracing is slow and not necessarily comprehensive in terms of the list of contacts, as well as hard to scale, implementation of a national digital contact tracing solution was considered.

Collaboration between Norwegian Institute of Public Health (NIPH) and Simula Research Laboratory (Simula) was set up to develop an efficient and scalable digital contact tracking solution. On the frontend, this solution would correspond to a mobile application (from here on, referred to as "mobile app" or "app") that could be installed on end user devices such as smartphones and wearables, run in the background without requiring any user interactions after registration, and continuously collect information about the device's own location as well as other devices in close proximity, using Global Positioning System (GPS) and Bluetooth (BT). Data from the mobile app would be collected centrally on the backend and analysed with an automated pipeline, allowing for the rapid generation of risk reports for every confirmed case. The complete system was named "Smittestopp".

The Smittestopp backend is one of the most crucial parts of the larger Smittestopp system, presented in Figure 3.1. It enables the ingestion and storage of data from the Smittestopp mobile app [15], which is detailed in Chapter 2, handles database and cloud operations for the automated processing and aggregation of these data by the Smittestopp analytics pipeline, which is detailed in Chapters 4 through 7, and interfaces with web applications, which were themselves outside the scope of the project on the Simula side.

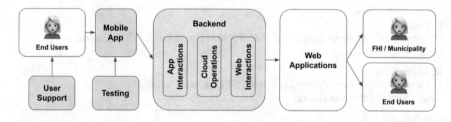

Fig. 3.1: Overview of the Smittestopp system, where coloured components indicate the scope of the technical solution developed by Simula. The focus of this chapter is in green.

The Smittestopp project had two main goals:

- An automatic solution for **contact tracing and notification** (*Varslingsløsning*) with a centralised architecture, for detecting those who have been in contact with

infected individuals. Support for an automated analytics pipeline, detecting and
tracing contacts between devices that have the mobile app installed.

- A solution for **aggregated statistics** (*Kunnskapsinnhenting*) that generates information on when and where contacts occured, how many people had encounters, and so on. Functionality was to be developed for tracing the spread of the
  pandemic throughout the country following national measures, via anonymised
  aggregations at the population level.

In this chapter, we give an overview of the backend solution put in place to address
and support these goals. Overall, the technical requirements from the Smittestopp
backend included both functional requirements for meeting the analytics needs and
nonfunctional requirements for fast and efficient data management, as well as for
protecting personal information. The development of the Smittestopp mobile app and
the analytics pipeline were covered in separate work packages and are elaborated
upon in different chapters of this book, namely, Chapters 2 and 6, respectively.

The remainder of this chapter is organised as follows: In Section 3.2, we describe
the technical implementation of the backend solution, including the architecture,
components, and end-to-end operations. In Section 3.3, we discuss how the implementation evolved over the course of five weeks, while being used nationally by
up to 1.5 million people, and we describe our experiences and lessons learned. We
conclude the chapter in Section 3.4. Readers who are interested in the technical details of our implementation are encouraged to continue reading through Section 3.2,
whereas readers who would like to focus on our lessons learned and discussions
can skip ahead to Section 3.3. The contents of Sections 3.2 and 3.3 can be studied
independently from one another.

3.2 Technical implementation

In this section, we provide a detailed description of the architecture, design, and
implementation of the Smittestopp backend, insofar as it was within the scope of the
project on the Simula side. We elaborate on the Smittestopp backend in the following manner: In Section 3.2.1, we reiterate the designated high level functionalities
required for the overall system. In Section 3.2.2, we provide a technical description
of the components and technologies that are employed in the Smittestopp backend
to support these functionalities. In Sections 3.2.3 to 3.2.5, we describe the role
played by the Smittestopp backend in delivering data from the mobile app to the web
applications in a usable manner, in line with the stated goals.

More specifically, in Section 3.2.3, we describe the first stage, denoted as app
interactions in Figure 3.1. This comprises a set of functions ranging from device
registration and deletion to authorisation, data upload, the handling of incoming
data with possible errors, and the transfer of data to the second phase of cloud-
based operations. In Section 3.2.4, we describe these cloud-based operations in
detail, including data ingestion and storage and running the analytics pipeline. In
Section 3.2.5, we elaborate on the higher-level services that the Smittestopp backend

provides to connected web applications in the form of the collection of endpoint queries. Further documentation related to the architecture and operations of the Smittestopp backend, please refer to the Smittestopp source code [21].

3.2.1 Required functionalities

3.2.1.1 Contact tracing and notification

One of the main goals of the Smittestopp system was to provide a centralised functionality for notifying people, in case they have been in contact with an infected individual. This is achieved through the use of an automated analytics pipeline detecting and tracing contacts between all devices that have the mobile app installed.

Summarised in Figure 3.2, the functionality works as follows: authorised accounts can use a web application to make queries such as list all close contacts of the user identified by phone number X, starting from a given date T, covering the past 14 days, where the threshold for a close contact is less than 2m for longer than 15 minutes. The query is serviced by the backend, and a response in the form of a report generated by the analytics pipeline is fed back to the web application.

See Section 3.2.5.1 for more details about the service we implemented to fulfil this functionality, and Chapters 4 through 6 for more details about the detection and reporting of contacts.

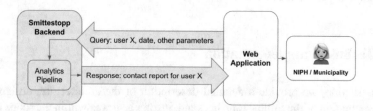

Fig. 3.2: High-level overview of the contact tracing functionality of the system, where coloured components indicate the scope of the backend solution.

3.2.1.2 Aggregated statistics

The second goal of the Smittestopp system was to provide additional information to support the tracing the of the spread of the pandemic throughout the country, especially following national measures. These are in the form of anonymised aggregations at the population level.

Summarised in Figure 3.3, the functionality works as follows: authorised accounts can use a web application to make queries such as list the number of contacts that have taken place in a specific Point of Interest (POI) (e.g. grocery stores), in a specific municipality (e.g. Oslo), on a given date T, with an hourly granularity. The query is serviced by the backend and an anonymised aggregate response, generated by the analytics pipeline, is fed back to the web application. The Points of Interest (POIs) can be any supported item, ranging from healthcare or education facilities to arts, entertainment, and culture or sports or commercial and residential areas [30]. The location of interest can be specified as a county (*fylke*), municipality (*kommune*), district (*bydel*), or basic statistical unit (*grunnkrets*)[1], or custom defined as an area polygon.

It should be noted here that only the NIPH and the government will have the clearance to run an aggregate statistics query. There are also constraints against running aggregate statistics in sparse spatiotemporal contexts, which carry the risk of revealing individual insights.

See Section 3.2.5.2 for more details about the service we implemented to fulfil this functionality, and Chapter 7 for more details about data aggregation and statistics (including privacy preserving techniques and anonymity).

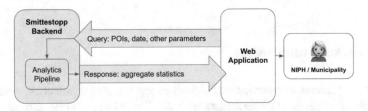

Fig. 3.3: High-level overview of the system's aggregated statistics functionality, where coloured components indicate the scope of the backend solution.

3.2.1.3 User data access

Additional functionality required of Smittestopp for transparency and privacy protection purposes was end user access to their own data. Support for this functionality was in the process of being developed.

Summarised in Figure 3.4, the functionality works as follows: any registered end user account can log in to https://helsenorge.no and browse all their GPS-based location data stored in the Smittestopp backend by date and time by using an Application Programming Interface (API) call. Users can also request an access log showing the details of all persons who have viewed their data including the legal means for doing so.

---

[1] For a full list of area identifiers in Norway, see [1, 26].

It should be noted here that only individual users will have the clearance to run this query, and they will only be able to retrieve their own data. Access to user data in this form and granularity is not available through any other service.

See Section 3.2.5.3 for more details about the service we began implementing to fulfil this functionality.

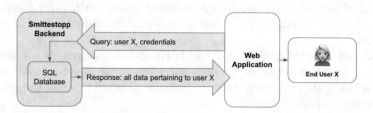

Fig. 3.4: High-level overview of the system's user data access functionality, where coloured components indicate the scope of the backend solution.

3.2.2 Backend components

Figure 3.5 presents an overview of the Smittestopp backend architecture, consisting of three main parts: (1) interactions with the Smittestopp mobile app, (2) cloud operations hosted on Microsoft Azure [10], and (3) interactions with a number of web applications maintained by NIPH and Helsenorge. Below, we provide a technical description of these components.

Note on sandboxing: To support the continuous development and testing of the Smittestopp backend solution, including after the national launch, and in a privacy-preserving manner, all Azure cloud resources (1 − 8) were duplicated into what are called development (`dev`) and production (`prod`) environments. These environments have different access rights, with corresponding mobile app versions targeting different registration services, and two completely different data sets being collected. The data in `dev`, incidentally much smaller in amount than in `prod`, are from informed volunteer testers, do not require anonymised processing, and can be used for research purposes. In addition to NIPH and Norwegian Health Network (NHN) [16] personnel, we recruited volunteers from Simula, along with any of their friends and family members who wanted to support the efforts, through internal campaigns (company-wide announcements) to contribute to the development process by testing different versions of the Smittestopp mobile app on their mobile devices. The valuable efforts from these volunteers complemented the more controlled testing approaches undertaken by the testing team (see Figure 3.1).

Note on performance monitoring: All backend components were instrumented with a monitoring tool called Azure Log Analytics [7]. This service is essentially in place for auditing (who accessed what, when, and why), troubleshooting, security

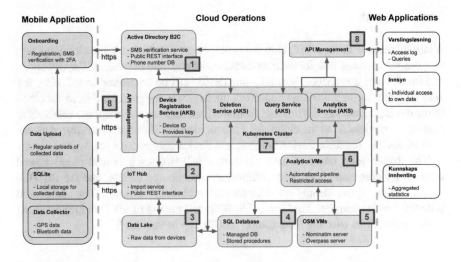

Fig. 3.5: Overview of the Smittestopp backend architecture. Coloured components indicate the scope of the technical solution developed by Simula.

monitoring, and performance monitoring purposes. The log analytics instance collects data from all Azure services, which is stored in a storage container designated by the account holder. Throughout Smittestopp's run, the log analytics instance was accessible only by NHN, and the developers and personnel to whom it explicitly extended access.

3.2.2.1 Active directory B2C

Azure Active Directory B2C (Azure AD B2C) provides Business-to-Consumer (B2C) identities as a service, where the customers can use their preferred social, enterprise, or local account identities to gain single sign-on access to applications and the APIs. It is a Customer Identity Access Management (CIAM) solution capable of supporting millions of users and billions of authentications per day. It takes care of the scaling and safety of the authentication platform, monitoring and automatically handling threats such as Denial of Service (DoS), password spraying, and brute force attacks [13].

All Azure services employed by the Smittestopp backend use the AD B2C enterprise identity service to provide single sign-on and multi-factor authentication. The component is denoted by the number 1 in Figure 3.5. We detail the use of Azure AD B2C in the context of cloud operations in Section 3.2.4.

3.2.2.2 IoT hub

Azure Internet of Things (IoT) Hub is a managed service hosted in the cloud that acts as a central message hub for bidirectional communication between IoT applications and the devices it manages. Virtually any device can be connected to IoT Hub. IoT Hub supports communications both from the device to the cloud and from the cloud to the device, as well as file uploads from devices, and request–response methods to control the devices from the cloud. IoT Hub monitoring allows the tracking of events such as device creations, device failures, and device connections [4].

The Smittestopp backend uses the Azure IoT Hub as a central cloud hosted solution for communication with Smittestopp mobile app clients, and the IoT Hub device registry as the identity provider for each mobile app instance. The component is denoted by the number 2 in Figure 3.5. We detail the use of IoT Hub in the context of the interactions with the Smittestopp mobile app in Section 3.2.3.

3.2.2.3 Data lake

Azure Data Lake Storage is a hyperscale repository for big data analytics workloads and a Hadoop Distributed File System (HDFS) for the cloud. It builds upon all features of Azure Blob Storage and adds a hierarchical namespace for efficient data access across large volumes of files. It imposes no fixed limits on file or account size. Azure Data Lake Storage uses Azure Active Directory (AD) for authentication and protects folders and files using Access Control Lists (ACLs). It allows for unstructured and structured data in their native formats and is tuned for massive throughput on large amounts of files [9].

GPS and BT data uploaded by Smittestopp mobile app clients to the Smittestopp backend passes through the Azure IoT Hub, and from there it is written in batches to a secure blob container in Azure Data Lake Storage Gen2. For troubleshooting purposes, an instance of Azure Search service was also created on top of the Azure Data Lake Storage container, which was designed to facilitate quick searches for event data belonging to a specific device. This component is denoted by the number 3 in Figure 3.5. We detail the use of Azure Data Lake in the context of cloud operations in Section 3.2.4.

3.2.2.4 SQL database

Azure SQL Database is based on SQL server database engine architecture that is adjusted for the cloud environment in order to ensure availability even in cases of infrastructure failure. The hyperscale service tier in is the newest service tier in the virtual core–based (vCore-based) purchasing model. It is a highly scalable storage and compute performance tier that leverages the Azure architecture to scale out storage and compute resources. The Azure SQL Database Hyperscale can scale up to a database of 100 TB, run on up to 80 vCores, and have up to five mirrored readable replicas. With replicas configured, the uptime SLA for the service is guaranteed at 99, 99% [8].

The Smittestopp backend uses an Azure SQL Database Hyperscale instance for most of its data analysis operations. This component is denoted by the number 4 in Figure 3.5. Data are ingested into the SQL Database from files in the Azure Data Lake. A major benefit of the hyperscale tier is that it has very short operational delays for reconfigurations and database restores, typically within 10 minutes, regardless of database size. SQL Database Hyperscale also supports index partitioning and compressed columnstore indexes, which provide an estimated compression of 10× on average, with a performance optimisation benefit as well. At peak usage, the Smittestopp database ran on 80 vCores with one readable replica and a database of 4 − 5 TB (compressed).

The Smittestopp database was completely locked down to allow access only to essential Azure services and application servers. All access was monitored by audit logs, and services only had access to the SQL functions they needed, besides two users with administrative access for deployment purposes, controlled by NHN. The component is denoted by the number 4 in Figure 3.5. We further elaborate on the use of the SQL Database in Section 3.2.4.

3.2.2.5 Data factory

Azure Data Factory is the main managed service in Azure for batch ingestion, and has a graphical interface for designing complex data flows and monitoring job executions [14].

The Smittestopp backend orchestrates data movement and performs data wrangling using Azure Data Factory. It uses Data Factory for loading data from Data Lake into Azure SQL Database, in addition to executing SQL stored procedures that perform additional data preparations after each batch ingestion. The data is not actually moved through the Data Factory service, which only executes commands against the underlying services. Azure Data Factory allows past jobs to be re-executed at the task level, which was an advantage for Smittestopp, since the system was not monitored 24/7. Data Factory jobs are run periodically, typically every hour. The service resides between the components denoted by the numbers 3 and 4 in Figure 3.5.

3.2.2.6 Stream analytics

Azure Stream Analytics is a serverless scalable Complex Event Processing (CEP) engine by Microsoft that enables users to develop and run real-time analytics on multiple streams of data from sources such as devices, sensors, web sites, social media, and other applications [12].

Within Smittestopp, the Azure Stream Analytics service was used initially to process incoming events from IoT Hub as data arrived, performing basic validation, filtration and pre-processing and continuously pushing data to the SQL Database.

The service was used during the first week of the launch, after which a decision was made to move to a batch ingestion process via Azure Data Lake Storage instead. The Stream Analytics job was abandoned after the Azure Data Factory jobs were running reliably. The switch took approximately one to two weeks and was accomplished with no downtime. The main reason for the switch was to improve the troubleshooting and end-to-end tracking of individual device events, which proved difficult with the Azure Stream Analytics service. We further detail the use of Stream Analytics in the context of cloud operations in Section 3.2.4 and discuss challenges related to data import, processing, and filtering in Section 3.3.

3.2.2.7 OSM VMs

Map matching involves combining GPS data with metadata from publicly available maps, in order to understand the kind of an environment in which a contact occured (e.g. inside a building, on public transportation, inside a private vehicle, outside), since this could impact the risk level of the contact, as well as the POIs around the contact (e.g. schools, grocery stores, public parks), which could allow for a more informed tracing of the performance of anti-pandemic measures. For the map matching purposes of the Smittestopp analytics pipeline (see Chapter 4 for details), we considered Google Maps [25], Azure Maps [6], and Open Street Maps (OSM) [19], before OSM was selected based on performance, metadata availability, and privacy requirements.

The Smittestopp backend hosts two OSM servers in each environment, (prod and dev). The OSM servers in the prod environment are only reachable from analytics Virtual Machines (VMs) in the prod environment. The servers in the prod environment use HTTPS. The corresponding Transport Layer Security (TLS) certificates contain only the names, and not specific IP addresses. This allows for future changes of the addresses.

- **OSM Nominatim:** This API is a tool to search OSM data by name and address (geocoding) and to generate synthetic addresses of OSM points (reverse geocoding) [28].
- **OSM Overpass:** This is a read-only API that serves up custom selected parts of the OSM map data. It acts as a database over the web: the client sends a query to the API and receives back the data set that corresponds to the query [29].

This component is denoted by the number 5 in Figure 3.5. We further elaborate on the use of the OSM servers in Section 3.2.4.

3.2.2.8 Analytics VMs

The Smittestopp backend hosts two VMs (Linux and Windows) in each environment, to support the development and execution of the Smittestopp analytics pipeline (Chapters 4 through 7). These machines have access to the SQL Database and the OSM VMs and are used to run the pipeline. The analytics VMs in the prod environment have restricted access. The component is denoted by the number 6 in Figure 3.5. We further elaborate on the use of the analytics VMs in Section 3.2.4.

3.2.2.9 Kubernetes cluster

Azure Kubernetes Service (AKS) is a cloud hosted service that manages Kubernetes and provides capabilities such as health monitoring, maintenance, and provisioning [5]. The Smittestopp backend uses an Azure Kubernetes cluster for hosting application services, where the following four dockerised services are deployed to AKS:

- **Device Registration Service:** This service handles device registration and consent revocation requests from the mobile app. Also shown are the clients for communicating with the following external services:

  – Microsoft Graph API (access point for information about Azure AD users)
  – IoT Hub (access point for information about devices)
  – SQL Database (GPS and BT data)

- **Deletion service:** This service is responsible for deleting data that is old or associated with users who have revoked their consent.
- **Query service:** This service handles requests from NIPH and Helsenorge. It uses Redis to queue analysis jobs that are processed by the analysis image when requested by NIPH.
- **Analytics service:** This service is responsible for identifying potential contacts between an infected individual and other application users over the time span requested by NIPH. The analysis service communicates with the other services through reads and writes to a Redis database.

The component is denoted by the number 7 in Figure 3.5. Relevant services are detailed in Sections 3.2.3, 3.2.4, and 3.2.5.

3.2.2.10 API endpoints

The Smittestopp backend serves three groups of endpoints, one for each of the following clients:

- Smittestopp mobile app
- NIPH web application
- Helsenorge web application

All Hypertext Transfer Protocol (HTTP) endpoints are managed in Azure API Management (APIM), which is configured via Terraform [3]. The details of the authentication processes vary with the endpoints that are called by the different clients. The mobile app endpoints are behind a Web Application Firewall (WAF), whereas the NIPH and Helsenorge endpoints are accessed directly in APIM (due to a lack of support for SSL client authorisation in WAF). A service prefix is added in APIM, namely, /fhi or /onboarding. Table 3.1 presents the list of endpoints. The APIM instances are denoted by the number 8 in Figure 3.5.

Type	Endpoint	Description
App	authentication	The app authenticates with a JavaScript Object Notation (JSON) web token from Azure AD B2C. Other endpoints authenticate with Hash-based Message Authentication Code (HMAC) signatures using the IoT Hub device ID and signing key.
	register new device	Registers a new device with IoT Hub and associates it with an existing user profile.
	revoke consent	Revokes permissions granted by a user. All data associated with the user will be deleted.
	request pin	Returns Personal Identification Number (PIN) codes for the given user.
	update birth year	Updates the registered birth year for the given user.
	request new bluetooth contact ids	Allocates and returns 10 new IDs for use as BT contact IDs.
FHI	lookup phone number	Requests contact tracing analysis to be performed for the given phone number.
	lookup result	Checks results from the contact tracing analysis for a given phone number. Returns results (200 OK) if the analysis is ready, or a not finished message (202 Accepted otherwise).
	access log	Returns the access log for a given user.
	egress	Returns the GPS events for a given user in a given time frame.
	lookup deleted numbers	Takes a list of phone numbers and returns the numbers not registered in the database.
Helsenorge	access log	Returns the access log for a given user.
	egress	Returns the GPS events for a given user in a given time frame.
	revoke consent	Revokes permissions granted by a user. All data associated with the user will be deleted.

Table 3.1: Smittestopp API endpoints.

3.2.3 Interactions with the mobile app

We now refer to the left part of Figure 3.5, which consists of the interactions between the Smittestopp backend and the Smittestopp mobile app. The components that are involved are numbered as 1 (AD B2C), 2 (IoT Hub), 7 (AKS), and 8 (APIM).

3.2.3.1 Key concepts

The key concepts for the interactions of the backend with the mobile app are as follows:

- A **device** is an instance of the Smittestopp mobile app that has a device ID in Azure IoT Hub and a phone number registered in Azure AD B2C.
- A **user** is defined as a phone number and can be tied to multiple devices.
- **Onboarding** is the process of guiding a new user through the registration process. This includes information about the Smittestopp mobile app, approval of the privacy policy, and entering the required information for registration.
- **Registration** is the process of signing up for Smittestopp using the mobile app. This process includes providing and verifying a phone number using a text message and providing and confirming the year of birth. The registration is described in more detail in Section 3.2.3.2.
- **Authentication** is the process of authenticating a user against one of the endpoints provided by the backend. In the Smittestopp mobile app, authentication is performed when registering a new user, logging in a previously registered user, and when revoking consent.
- **Deletion** is the process of revoking consent for the collection of data and deleting any stored information about the user. In addition to automatic deletion, manual deletion can be undertaken by the user, either in the mobile app or in the web application through the user data access service (*Innsyn*).

3.2.3.2 Registration

Following mobile app installation, users are prompted to undertake SMS verification. Users are onboarded by registering their phone number and authenticating their identities with a B2C login in the app. User profiles and corresponding devices are managed by Azure AD B2C and IoT Hub, respectively.

User accounts live in Azure AD B2C, a different tenant from the main deployment for dev and prod. This is where phone numbers (as users) and device IDs (as groups) and their associations (group membership) are recorded. The B2C HTML templates are uploaded with Terraform. The B2C custom policy files, which specify how apps can be authenticated, are uploaded via the Azure B2C Identity Experience Framework. The policy files are different for dev and prod (only in some allowed URLs and tenant IDs) and are uploaded via the upload custom policy link on the Identify Experience Framework page. Login is disabled for prod.

3.2.3.3 Data upload

After registration with a phone number and SMS verification, the user receives a unique ConnectionDeviceID from the Azure IoT Hub registry. This ID is later used to identify the user whenever data are uploaded, and it identifies data from a specific user in the database. When the mobile app uploads data, it identifies itself using the `ConnectionDeviceID` and then sends the payload, which consists of a JSON document with GPS and BT events to the IoT Hub HTTP endpoint.

3.2.3.4 Deletion

The Smittestopp privacy policy indicates that databases that contain private information, such as phone numbers and GPS (location) data, must be deletable upon request by end users. The policy for deletion can be summarised as follows:

1. All GPS (location) and BT (contact) data will be deleted automatically, 30 days after upload.
2. A user can ask for their data to be deleted at any time.
3. A user who is inactive for more than seven days will be deleted, including all of the user's data.

Deletion according to item 1 is performed by a stored procedure in the SQL Database that runs every night and deletes all data older than 30 days and any other data marked for deletion.

User-initiated deletion according to item 2 is slightly more complex, since it involves deletion from both the B2C and SQL Database. When the user presses the Delete button in the mobile app, the user's device IDs are immediately dissociated from the user's phone number, the user's phone number is deleted from AD B2C, and all device IDs are marked for deletion in AD B2C. These device IDs are immediately unregistered from IoT Hub. At this point, the user's GPS and BT data still remain in the SQL Database, but cannot be linked to a phone number and thus cannot be returned via the internal or external APIs, which operate solely based on phone numbers (*Varslingsløsning, Innsyn*). The remaining data will be deleted as part of the nightly run of the stored procedure in SQL. To avoid the delayed import of data associated with deleted device IDs, after a device ID has been shown to have no data in the SQL Database for multiple days, it is finally removed from AD B2C.

Deletion according to item 3 is the most complex, since IoT Hub does not reliably provide information about the last activity from a device. This issue is resolved by checking the last time a user wrote data in the SQL Database and marking the user for deletion if the user has not written data in the last seven days. This procedure was later updated by introducing a heartbeat from the mobile app to the backend, which can be used to check the time of last activity.

The SQL Database (but not B2C) is backed up using standard cloud database backup strategies. According to item 1, backups must expire in at most 30 days. Data deleted according to items 2 or 3 are not deleted immediately from backups. However, the phone numbers are not backed up and cannot be restored, only anonymous device ID data can, which cannot be extracted from the system except by the database administrators. No database backup restoration occurs during Smittestopp's operation, but the described protection against delayed import also protects against temporarily restoring data from backups. If a backup restores data from a deleted device ID, the deletion procedure will still be running and it will be deleted again upon the next deletion procedure, within 24 hours. This means that, to preserve the deletion policy, database backups older than the deletion recheck window (between two and seven days, according to the configuration) cannot be restored. In summary,

1. Previously deleted data restored from a backup can never be accessed via APIs because it cannot be reassociated with a phone number.
2. Previously deleted data will be deleted again immediately upon the next nightly deletion procedure, since the device ID will still be registered for deletion.

3.2.4 Cloud operations

We now refer to the central part of Figure 3.5, consisting of the Smittestopp backend operations taking place in the Azure cloud. Core components 2 − 7 are involved.

3.2.4.1 Data ingest and storage

Data ingest and storage refers to the operations of components 2 and 3, where the data uploaded by mobile app clients are ingested by the Smittestopp backend. Mobile app clients send event data to the public IoT Hub endpoint, authenticating by certificate. Event data in IoT Hub is considered a *Message*, and IoT Hub adds to each message payload a section with IoT Hub metadata, including the ConnectionDeviceID which identifies each unique device and will be used in the database will be used as the device identifier across event data. Event messages are of two types, GPS or BT, with each message containing an array of multiple events.

IoT Hub is configured with four partitions that split incoming data into four parallel flows and a message routing rule that writes all incoming messages into 10 MB uncompressed chunks to Azure Data Lake Storage. In addition, for the first weeks, a streaming endpoint was configured in IoT Hub to which Azure Stream Analytics subscribed for real-time events, which was later abandoned for a pure Data Lake Storage–oriented architecture (see Section 3.2.2.6 for details).[2]

In the Azure Data Lake, filenames are created according to the pattern yyyy/mm/dd/hh/yyyy-mm-dd-hh-mm-partitionID.json, where each file corresponds to one 10MB chunk. This naming scheme supports up to four files per minute when including a partitionID from zero to three. If the injection rate leads to the creation of more than four files per minute, a sequence number is added to the

---

[2] Stream Analytics was configured with an input from IoT Hub and outputs for each staging table in the SQL Database. The Stream Analytics Query Language (SAQL) query undertaking the transformation from input to output, mapped each field from the input JSON to the output database table columns, validating the datatype, length, and filters for special characters. In addition, it performed a streaming aggregation on each event array using the GetArrayElement function within the execution context of the defined time window.

filename. Data Lake is configured to delete data older than seven days. At peak load, the Smittestopp data lake had up to about 1, 500 individual 10 MB files an hour.

3.2.4.2 SQL database operations

Schema: Table 3.2 presents a list of tables common for the dev and prod environments.

Table	Description
dbo.agg_gpsevents	Aggregated table
dbo.btevents	BT pairing events
dbo.dluserdatastaging	Device information
dbo.gpsevents	GPS events
dbo.grunnkrets	Geospatial lookups using the geography datatype
dbo.uuid_activity	For tracking users who were inactive for 7+ days
dbo.uuid_id	Supporting table for Universally Unique Identifier (UUID) <-> internal ID mapping

Table 3.2: Smittestopp main SQL database tables.

Import: Every hour, Azure Data Factory triggers an import job that imports data from Azure Data Lake to the SQL Database. This job is set up as a pipeline with the following steps:

1. Four parallel tasks (ADSLIMPORTER) import files from each of the four partitions from the last hour into the table DLUSERDATASTAGING in the SQL Database. The import procedure extracts UUID, platform, appversion, osversion and model from the JSON document and stores them in individual columns. The event payload is stored as an unprocessed JSON in a separate column. The name of the source file is included in the table so that all data can be traced back to the file of origin. Each tasks is authenticated using SQL stored credentials mapped to an Azure service principal with the exact permissions to execute the import task.

2. When ADSLIMPORTER is done, another two parallel tasks start. These are the BTIMPORTER and GPSIMPORTER procedures for importing BT and GPS events, respectively. These procedures process the information imported by ADSLIMPORTER in Step 1, as follows:

   a. GPSIMPORTER imports all the GPS data from the unprocessed JSON column to the GPSEVENTS table.

   b. BTIMPORTER updates the UUID_ID table so that UUIDs are mapped to internal keys and imports all the BT data from the unprocessed JSON column to the BTEVENTS table. Then it updates the UUID_ACTIVITY table, which stores the

time of last activity for all UUIDs. This is used by the deletion routines to
delete data from devices that have been inactive for more than seven days.

3. The last step is the execution of the AGGREGATOR procedure to populate the
   AGG_GPSEVENTS table according to the following criteria:

   a. Downsample the GPS events to only include one GPS event every 10 seconds
      for each UUID.
   b. Execute the STWITHIN procedure to carry out a geospatial lookup of the correct
      grunnkrets[3] for each GPS event.
   c. Round all GPS coordinates to two decimal places (both latitude and longitude).
   d. Remove duplicates.

Procedures and functions: The SQL Database has stored procedures and functions for managing access to user data. These allow database users (e.g. AKS) to
retrieve processed versions of the raw data, since the database tables cannot be
queried directly.

3.2.4.3 Analytics pipeline

The Smittestopp analytics pipeline is executed by running the Dockerised analytics
service deployed on AKS (component 7 in Figure 3.5).

Configuration: The list of configurations for the pipeline can be passed as a
JSON file to the Docker container, or as environment variables. For instance, the
Smittestopp backend has support for setting OSM endpoints using environment variables (CORONA_OVERPASS_ENDPOINT and CORONA_NOMINATIM_ENDPOINT). DNS
names, instead of IP addresses are used.

Database access: Credentials for connecting to the SQL Database are provided
as configuration parameters. Since the database can be accessed only from within
a VPN, the analytics service can only be run from within the Smittestopp cloud
infrastructure (e.g. Analytics VMs, denoted by 6 in Figure 3.5). Data in the SQL
Database can only be accessed through predefined procedures and functions, as
described in Section 3.2.4.2.

More details about the Smittestopp analytics pipeline are provided in Chapters 4
through 7.

3.2.5 Interactions with web applications

The general goals of the Smittestopp system listed in Section 3.1 and the particular
functionalities required of the Smittestopp backend listed in Section 3.2.1 result
in three services that access the Smittestopp APIs: contact tracing and notification

---

[3] The *grunnkrets* is the basic statistical unit defined by Statistics Norway [26].

(*Varslingsløsning*), aggregated statistics (*Kunnskapsinnhenting*), and user data access (*Innsyn*). These services are described below, while the APIs endpoints are listed in Section 3.2.2.10.

3.2.5.1 Contact tracing and notification service (*Varslingsløsning*)

Contact tracing with Smittestopp is performed by NIPH rather than by individuals, as is the case for solutions based on Google/Apple Exposure Notifications (GAEN). With Smittestopp, an employee at NIPH regularly receives a list of infected individuals from the Norwegian Surveillance System for Communicable Diseases (MSIS), which includes their name, Social Security number, and phone number. The Smittestopp API (see Section 3.2.2.10) is then used to look up close contacts for each individual, based on the phone number provided. The lookup process works as follows:

1. NIPH makes a call to the `lookup phone number` endpoint with the phone number of a person who has tested positive for COVID-19 as input.
2. Based on the request, an analysis job is scheduled by creating a record in a Redis database.
3. A link to an endpoint for receiving the result is returned to the caller. This endpoint is called by the NIPH web application until it receives response `200`, which indicates that the request is complete.
4. The analytics service picks jobs from the queue in the Redis database and performs a contact analysis.
5. When the analytics job is complete, the result (list of contacts) is stored in JSON format in the Redis object under the result key.
6. The analysis report is returned to the NIPH web application (see Step 3). From the report, NIPH can notify those who are likely to have been in contact with the infected individual during the period specified in the request.

The actual notification of those who have been in close contact with an infected individual is carried out manually, where a human verifies that all the data are correct and then sends a text message to everyone who have been exposed to infection. The text message warns about potential infection and informs the individual about recommended steps for testing. The long-term plan was to eliminate the manual steps and automate lookup and notification, but this work was never completed. This service does not have any publicly exposed endpoints.

3.2.5.2 Aggregated statistics service (*Kunnskapsinnhenting*)

To support mathematical modelling and epidemiological studies, a service for extracting statistics regarding the pandemic from the Smittestopp data was in development, but never fully implemented. The idea was to provide statistics based on the collected data, such as where infections are occurring (e.g. regions of Norway, different POIs, home vs. work), the current infection rate (increasing, constant, or decreasing), and the average number of close contacts per person. See Chapter 7 for more details.

3.2.5.3 User data access service (*Innsyn*)

For Smittestopp to be compliant with the General Data Protection Regulation (GDPR), it must provide a way for individuals to access any of their personal data used in any way by the system. Therefore, a right of access service is a mandatory part of the Smittestopp architecture. This is implemented as a web service where Smittestopp users can log in and browse all of their GPS-based location data stored in Smittestopp by date and time, using the `egress` call (see Section 3.2.2.10). Furthermore, users can request the access log showing the details of all persons who have viewed their data, including the legal means for doing so. The service was part of `Helsenorge.no` and users where authenticated using ID-porten, a common login solution for public services in Norway. The right of access service, as described above, was never fully operational due to performance issues. An asynchronous solution where a user requests data for later delivery was planned but never implemented.

3.3 Experience: Challenges and lessons learned

In this section, we focus on our experiences with the development and implementation of the Smittestopp backend solution, and describe our lessons learned, along with general insights.

3.3.1 Distributed versus centralised architecture

As indicated in Section 3.1, the Smittestopp backend had a design requirement to run in a centralised manner, relying on cloud components and operations such as a centrally managed data storage, server-side execution of an automated analytics pipeline, and the externally triggered generation of contact and statistics reports by public authorities. This requirement was in line with the intended twofold purpose of the overall system, that is, simultaneous contact tracing and aggregated statistics generation.

During the project's development and launch, as well as after its recall, there were many discussions, both internal and external, regarding the viability of a distributed solution (as opposed to a centralised one). Shortly before the launch of the Smittestopp system, the GAEN initiative demonstrated that a distributed, purely BT-based approach could be used for individualised contact tracing, potentially serving as a more privacy-preserving and secure alternative to centralised solutions.

However, with respect to the requirements mentioned in Section 3.1, storing data only locally on end user devices, in a fully distributed system, could be highly impractical for a number of reasons. Including concerns regarding the data volume, processing time, and network transactions, two fundamental global challenges were identified: the impossibility of listing second-level contacts and the impossibility of generating nationwide aggregated statistics.

In a distributed scheme, an end user device can, based on its location, create a list of devices with which it has had direct contact (along with the corresponding location of each contact). However, listing second-level contacts would require more information located on other devices. Second, generating aggregated statistics based on queries such as 'list all contacts that have happened yesterday at shopping mall X' would be a huge and costly operation, requiring communication with all active devices in the system and requesting information on whether they were in the given location at the given time. Therefore, after evaluating these challenges together with the initial system requirements and the need for fast deployment, the Smittestopp backend development was continued in pursuit of a centralised solution.

The security and privacy assessments regarding a centralised solution were also supported by the Ministry of Health and Care Services [17], and it was pointed out that the management of personal information was subject to *Personvernforordningen* articles 6 and 9, such that the overall gain from the system outweighed the potential privacy concerns.

Considering other contact tracing solutions, we see that, as of May 2020, 16 countries [18] had launched or had in development a system based on a centralised approach, including COVIDSafe (Australia), StopCovid (France), Trace Together (Singapore), and HaMagen (Israel), whereas 25 countries used systems based on a decentralised approach, including COVID Alert (Canada), Ketju (Finland), Corona-Warn-App (Germany), and NHS COVID-19 App (UK).[4] With the launch of GAEN, many countries decided to abandon their own solutions in favour of a GAEN-based approach. For several countries, such as the United Kingdom, this meant switching from a centralised to a decentralised solution.

In Norway, discussions were held regarding the adoption of a GAEN-based approach for contact tracing, along with the development a separate solution for generating nationwide aggregated statistics, thereby splitting the desired functionalities into two distinct systems [20, 2].

Mobile apps for digital contact tracing have also been discussed in the previous chapter, under Section 2.2. We discuss privacy- and security-related aspects in Section 3.3.4.

---

[4] For a comprehensive list of contact tracing solutions around the globe, readers are referred to [22].

3.3.2 Data processing

As described in Section 3.2.1, multiple functionalities were required from the Smittestopp backend with respect to data processing. Each of these imposed different demands on the backend solution and gave rise to various challenges. Below, we focus on the functionalities addressed by the contact tracing and notification service (*Varslingsløsning*) and the aggregated statistics service (*Kunnskapsinnhenting*) as particular examples and discuss some of the data processing challenges we have addressed, along with our experiences.

Functionality 1 (contact tracing using GPS data): The first functionality aims to find those who have potentially been in contact with infected individuals, thus having a risk of being infected themselves. Assuming accurate GPS positions, finding who has been in contact with whom at any given point is supposedly an easy task. The task translates to finding the trajectory of an infected individual and then finding others whose trajectories intersected with this trajectory, that is, those who were at the same location at the same point in time. As shown in Figure 3.6, this means following the red trajectory (infected person) and finding all positions where it intersects with another trajectory, within an allowed distance threshold, such as the blue trajectory (of other person). A very simplified pseudocode, checking everything in a straightforward manner and aiming to solve the intersection problem solely by an SQL query is shown in Figure 3.7, where `infected` and `others` represent tables including GPS data.

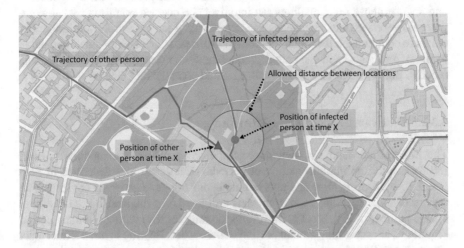

Fig. 3.6: Identifying GPS intersections: for every point on the trajectory of the infected person, find the matching positions of other persons within a distance (radius) X. Map from https://www.norgeskart.no.

Functionality 2 (deriving aggregated statistics): The second functionality aims at generating overall population statistics on how people move and how the disease

```
SELECT (relevant information from) others
FROM infected JOIN others ON
    infected.id = <ID of infected person> AND
    infected.id != others.id AND
WHERE
    infected.location WITHIN (others.location + <allowed distance>) AND
    infected.time BETWEEN <date_from> AND <date_to> AND
    others.time BETWEEN <date_from> AND <date_to> AND
    infected.time OVERLAP others.time
```

Fig. 3.7: Simplified query to find GPS intersections, given the ID of infected person, a threshold for the allowed distance, and a time range in the form of date_from and data_to.

spreads. As an example of aggregated statistics, let us assume that we need to find all encounters that happened within a given area, defined by a polygon, corresponding to a Norwegian geographical area unit called *grunnkrets* (the basic statistical unit in Norway, providing a stable and coherent geographical identification). To give an idea of the complexity involved, Figure 3.8 shows how the city of Oslo is divided into *delbydeler*, the statistical unit above the *grunnkrets*, each consisting of several *grunnkretser*. In total, there are about 14,000 *grunnkretser* in Norway. Thus, for each *grunnkrets*, we should be able to find all BT pairings that happened within the polygon defining this area and can match the time of the contact to the requested time interval (Figure 3.9).

Overview of challenges: Given the simplicity of the pseudocode in Figures 3.7 and 3.9, the above functionalities can intuitively be deemed relatively easy to compute. However, various challenges and complicating factors arise, even in the dev database containing a few hundred thousand entries, which is very small compared to the prod database in the actual production system containing millions of data records. Below, we discuss these challenges and complicating factors.

3.3.2.1 Date ranges and columnstore storage

The Smittestopp database contains entries from a relatively long time interval (30 days, after the implementation of periodic data deletion as described in Section 3.2.3.4). Storing large amounts of data in one big table generally constitutes an overhead, and, depending on how the data are stored, one might also need to access a large number of disk blocks. However, searching for data within a limited period requires us to access only a small portion of the entries. Bearing in mind that contact tracing typically requires going back only a few days (14 or, more commonly, seven days) and that our queries usually have a granularity of days, we implemented an optimisation in the form of *columnstore* storage, to increase efficiency. Columnstore indexing provides the physical storage of data that is already grouped by day. The speed of our queries can thus be increased.

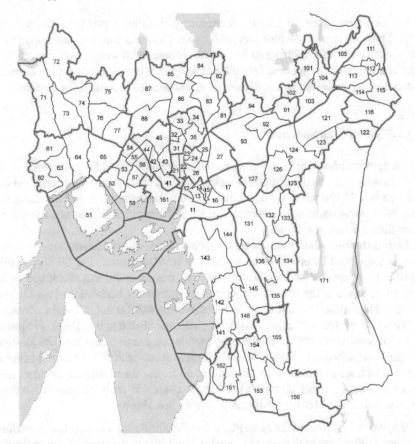

Fig. 3.8: Norway has many *grunnkretser*. The image above shows how Oslo alone is divided into *delbydeler*, each consisting of multiple *grunnkretser* (map from https://no.wikipedia.org/wiki/Delbydeler_i_Oslo).

```
SELECT (encounter data from both tables)
FROM gps-events a JOIN bt-events b ON
    a.uuid = b.uuid AND
    b.pairedtime BETWEEN a.timefrom AND a.timeto
WHERE
    a.location WITHIN <polygon>
    b.pairedtime BETWEEN <date_from> AND <date_to>
```

Fig. 3.9: Simplified query combining GPS and BT data to find all encounters inside a `polygon` within a time range given by `date_from` and `date_to`.

3.3.2.2 Inaccurate GPS measurements

As a technology, GPS itself has limited accuracy [24]. This is further complicated by variations in the location accuracy as reported by different end user device platform and models (see Section 2.6.2 for a discussion of location services in Android and iOS). Thus, we cannot test for exact position matches in our queries and must allow for slack. This is shown in Figure 3.6, where we search for a match within a certain diameter around a given point. Overall, not being able to check for position equality but, rather, for inclusion within a given area, our queries become more complex.

3.3.2.3 Timestamp matching

Clock synchronisation: In a perfect world, all devices would keep the exact same time. However, in practice, different clocks can be off by up to several seconds, which must be considered when we query for matching timestamps. Thus, matching the time between two entries translates to checking whether their timestamps overlap by more than a certain threshold.

Encounter duration: From a contact tracing viewpoint, an encounter must exceed a certain duration threshold to be counted as a valid contact. For GPS data, this threshold was defined as 15 minutes, meaning that an additional check had to be performed to see if the sum of the individual encounters between devices D1 and D2 lasted more than this threshold, before declaring that D1 and D2 had a contact.

Timestamps from location entries: A challenge related to timekeeping in terms of the GPS entries is that the Smittestopp mobile app can only register GPS location information (latitude and longitude) in the form of events with timefrom and timeto fields, which are not necessarily the same at all times. When calculating encounter durations, the following approach is taken. A contact is reported only if the total encounter duration exceeds the threshold mentioned above.

- If a device is staying in the same place, and the Smittestopp mobile app is reading many GPS events with the same location but different timestamps, the app itself will merge the records, keeping the location and the timefrom timestamp from the first data record and the timeto timestamp from the last data record in the series. Thus, the difference between the timeto and timefrom fields can be used to indicate the total time the device has spent in the given location and can be directly added to the total encounter duration.

- If the device is moving, the GPS events read by the app will have timefrom=timeto, with different locations indicated by consecutive records. Thus, if a device is moving through points P1 and P2, which are identified as part of an intersecting path (two devices are moving together on this path), the time between the timefrom timestamp of point P1 and the timefrom timestamp of the consecutive point P2 can be added to the total encounter duration.

3.3.2.4 Calculating speed and distance

From an analytics perspective, trajectory calculation also involves determining the mode of transport for nonstationary devices (see Chapter 4 for details on the

Smittestopp analytics pipeline). However, in order to establish a mode of transport, information about the speed is necessary. Various reports indicate that the estimated speed reported by the built-in GPS of end user devices such as smartphones, tablets, and smartwatches are highly inaccurate. Therefore, we needed to calculate the speed of the moving devices ourselves, based on the location and timestamps indicated by consecutive GPS records (using the `lag` function).

3.3.2.5 Calculating distance on a sphere

Due to the curvature of the earth, using the Pythagorean theorem [31] to calculate the distance between two pairs of coordinates is not 100% accurate. As a remedy, the Haversine distance [27] can be used to find the great circle distance between two points on a sphere, given their longitudes and latitudes. However, computing the Haversine distance is a complex and costly operation. In the Smittestopp backend, we implemented a simplified version of this distance as a trade-off between accuracy and processing costs. The simplification produces minimal errors, since, for our use case, the distances involved are relatively short.

Given that the diameter of the Earth is 12, 742, 016 metres, the distance between two points can be calculated as follows:

```
distance between points A (@LatA, @LongA) and B (@LatB, @LongB) =
    12742016 * asin(min(sqrt((sin(radians(@LatB - @LatA)/2)
    * sin(radians(@LatB - @LatA)/2)
    + cos(radians(@LatA))
    * cos(radians(@LatB))
    * sin(radians(@LongB - @LongA)/2)
    * sin(radians(@LongB - @LongA)/2)))))
```

This trade-off formula provides sufficiently accurate distances, but it is a question of whether the computation is still overkill. Most of the distances we calculate are rather short (with only a small error due to the Earth's curvature), and the accuracy of the GPS records themselves are also questionable. Thus, in a future system similar to Smittestopp, the differences between a plain Pythagorean calculation and a Haversine calculation, in terms of accuracy versus computing costs, should be investigated more closely.

3.3.2.6 Location pre-filtering

To reduce the number of entries in the JOIN operation when we search for matches within an area, we can pre-filter entries, that is, group them per unit bounding box of 1 kilometre, with respect to their latitude and longitude.

The distance between two consecutive degrees of latitude is constant (111.045 kilometres everywhere on Earth):

```
latitude between <latitude> ± (1 / 111.045)
```

The distance between two consecutive degrees of longitude is not constant (the distances are smaller the further away they are from the equator):

```
longitude between <longitude> ± (1 / (111.045 * cos(radians(latitude))))
```

3.3.2.7 Trajectory segmentation

Taking into account all the features of our database, it was clear from the start that the queries from Figures 3.7 and 3.9 might not be straightforward. However, tuning such queries on the dev database is still possible with return times in seconds or minutes, that is, seemingly within the operational thresholds of a normal web application. On the other hand, going from the dev database to the prod database (number of database records on the order of one hundred million, versus the meagre one hundred thousand in dev) leads to new challenges.

On the largest instance on Azure, with 80 vCores, such queries took days to finish, such that we could not depend on the database to run queries that were too complex over too large a time span over too large a geographical area. This demonstrated the need for a distributed computing approach, where we would divide our tasks into smaller subtasks, and assign these to different processors or machines.

After several optimisations were tested, the final deployed solution would divide a user's trajectory into smaller segments of geographical areas (bounding boxes) and time intervals, as depicted in Figure 3.10. To offload the database server, user data from these bounding boxes and time intervals would be sent to the analytics pipeline (described in Chapter 6) for further fine-grained processing.

3.3.2.8 Data sanity checks

Importing data from millions of devices outside one's control naturally resulted in a certain number of invalid data samples in our database. Among the samples collected, we observed both erroneous timestamps (date and/or time) and erroneous GPS locations. For instance, numerous records had timestamps indicating dates long before or after the period the Smittestopp system had been running. There could have been several reasons for this, but since we had no way of knowing the correct timestamps, such records were removed. Additionally, we also observed anomalous latitude and longitude values, where devices known to be in Norway had sent GPS records indicating locations far outside the country. Again, there could have been different reasons, such as hardware or operating system problems, GPS jammers in certain areas, and so forth. Nevertheless, these records were also removed from the database. To handle such cases, data sanity checks during data import were used, and sanity check operations were added to the mobile app at a later stage, to avoid sending erroneous data in the first place.

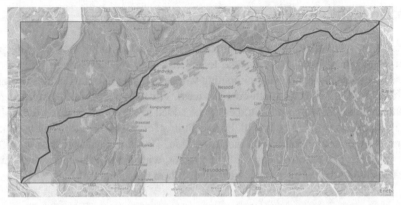

(a) Searching an entire trajectory within one operation, yielding a huge area over an entire period.

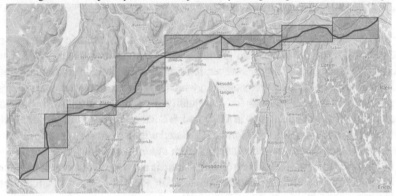

(b) Dividing the trajectory into multiple smaller segments, greatly reducing the search area, with a shorter, distinct time interval for each segment.

Fig. 3.10: Sample search area when an infected individual travels from Drammen to Lillestrøm.

3.3.2.9 Database schema updates

To optimise certain data operations and calculations that were run multiple times within the analytics pipeline, we traded off storage for faster data analysis. For instance, we introduced the notion of precalculated values during the data import stage. For a given device, these include the speed and distance between the current and previous locations, as well as an associated *grunnkrets* for every GPS entry, depending on the latitude and longitude. To store these values, database tables were augmented with additional columns and new tables were constructed to optimise operations for various specialised queries – to a large degree breaking traditional database normalisation rules, but yielding considerable gains in terms of processing speed.

3.3.2.10 Moving operations to end user devices

Another way of distributing the processing load is to move some of the pre-calculations and data sanity checks to the end user devices, which collectively constitute a far more powerful computing source than any of our machines in Azure (which were 1.5 million multi-core devices). For example, a device's speed and distance between two points could easily be added to the computation in the mobile app before data are sent to the IoT Hub, avoiding frequently repeated and computationally expensive operations on the server side. The same could be done with data sanity checks. In the final stages of the project, with the system being shut down, these tasks were delayed and now remain as future suggestions.

3.3.2.11 Manual versus automatic tracing

There is no doubt that digital solutions allowing for the automatic and large-scale execution of certain analyses can greatly assist organisations such as NIPH with their efforts in contact tracing. However, it is important to note that the quality of an analysis is never better than the dataset on which it is based. In the previous sections, we pointed out several sources for low-quality data, including but not limited to timestamp errors or inaccuracy in GPS and BT samples. Some of the challenges associated with low-quality data can be alleviated with certain system optimisations, and some cannot. Therefore, the analyses from systems such as Smittestopp should not be assumed to be completely error-free. There is also a greater, more fundamental challenge for such solutions: people can turn off their devices or disable contact tracing apps, meaning there are no data at all.

There were several occasions during the testing period when Simula was informed by NIPH that the automatic system had detected more encounters than the manual tracing process, which was encouraging. However, digital contact tracing solutions should not be perceived as complete alternatives for replacing manual procedures, but, rather, as supplementary mechanisms to support the existing systems. For a more detailed discussion of digital versus manual tracing, see Chapter 6.

3.3.3 Cloud optimisations

Some of the challenges we faced through the development of the Smittestopp backend concern the efficient use of the cloud components described in Section 3.2.2. Below, we provide examples for two such aspects.

3.3.3.1 Handling data import

As mentioned in Section 3.2.4.1, the Azure Stream Analytics service was used in the first weeks of development for processing incoming events, for basic validation, filtration, and pre-processing, and for pushing data to the SQL Database. The service was later abandoned for a pure Data Lake Storage–oriented architecture with batch ingestion.

One of the biggest challenges causing this change was that the Smittestopp mobile app instances on some smartphones were sending the same event data over and over again, while others were sending data at very high frequencies (up to one event per second), which needed to be filtered out early in the data processing pipeline.[5] These filters required database lookups that are better to implement in set-oriented batch processes. The shift from the Azure Stream Analytics service also improved the troubleshooting and end-to-end tracking of individual device events overall.

3.3.3.2 Managing load on components

One example related to managing the operational load on the backend components was the need to optimise the use of the OSM servers and, more specifically, to prevent the Overpass API from becoming a bottleneck during the execution of the Smittestopp analytics pipeline.

The background to this problem is that we were seeing a bottleneck in the calls to this server while querying POIs for a given trajectory. The initial implementation tried to utilise the server better by sending many small requests in parallel, but this was perceived as causing a bottleneck. To address this problem, we introduced an alternative code path in the analytics service (AKS) that tries to exploit the fact that the bounding boxes for the points along a trajectory will have considerable overlap. This way, for a typical trajectory, the number of requests were reduced to one. Further work would still be needed to handle very long trajectories.

3.3.4 Ethical, privacy and security aspects

The use of GPS and BT data in association with user IDs carries the risk of revealing personal information. However, one of the goals of the Smittestopp backend is to inform persons if they have been in contact with an infected individual, necessitating an ID in one form or another to be stored in the system. Therefore, a number of measures were implemented in the Smittestopp backend to make the system as

---

[5] On the mobile app side, bugs in the development of the software could lead to the same data being sent over and over again, whereas the frequency of sending data had inherent limitations and differences with respect to different platforms (Android vs. iOS). From an analytics perspective, it was also a matter of discussion *how* the local data on the smartphones should be pre-processed before being sent to the database in the backend.

secure and privacy preserving as possible. In this section, we elaborate on some of these measures and associated challenges.

3.3.4.1 Overview of security measures

The Smittestopp backend relies on the Microsoft Azure cloud infrastructure at an enterprise service tier, thereby inheriting all generic security measures available for business solutions. All Azure services employed by the Smittestopp backend use the Azure AD B2C enterprise identity service to provide single sign-on and multi-factor authentication.

Data in transit: The Smittestopp backend uses encrypted communications in all mobile app and web interactions (see Sections 3.2.3 and 3.2.5), firewalls in authentication processes and hidden APIs (see Section 3.2.2.10), and HTTPS access to all servers with TLS certificates (see Section 3.2.2.7).

Data at rest: All storage in Azure SQL Database, storage containers, and so on, as well as the respective backups are secured with encryption at rest, and the encryption keys are stored in the customer key vault service. The backend also employs multilevel access, limited user groups (depending on the level of authorisation), and cross-organisation data splitting (according to the scope of authority).

3.3.4.2 Data anonymisation

Data anonymisation refers to the removal of personally identifiable information from data sets, so that the individuals the data describes remain anonymous [23]. Within the Smittestopp system, all operations after the registration are based on devices (not users) and are undertaken through the use of non–human-readable UUIDs.

In the Smittestopp backend, with the exception of AD (component 1 in Figure 3.5), none of the components use any identifier that can be associated with an individual or phone number. All data operations within the backend (components 2 – 8 in Figure 3.5, including IoT Hub, Data Lake, and SQL Database) use the device handle UUID, as mentioned above. AD lookups in the prod environment are subject to extremely tight restrictions and strict auditing, with no more than two people in the entire project having access to the directory.

Although it is not possible to run a completely privacy-preserving operation within the centralised confines of our operation (see Sections 3.1 and 3.2.1 to review the design specifications, and Section 3.3.1 for a general discussion of centralised vs. distributed architectures), a certain level of privacy has been ensured in this regard. We refer readers to Chapter 7 for a detailed discussion of anonymity within the context of aggregated statistics.

3.3.4.3 Data storage

From the start of the project, it was a priority that the physical storage of any user data associated with Smittestopp complied with the jurisdiction of the European GDPR. In this regard, all Smittestopp backend components resided in Europe since the first day. Major components such as Data Lake and SQL Database were located in Norway from the beginning. However, at the time we went into production, Microsoft's data centre in Norway had just recently opened, and a number of Azure services were not yet available in Norway. Some components, such as the IoTHub and Stream Analytics engine, were located in the Northern Europe data centre (Ireland) for a few weeks. Afterwards, in the second phase, the backend was reconfigured, and most of the services were relocated to Norway. During the reconfiguration, we also scrapped Stream Analytics and moved to a data load from file approach, as mentioned in Sections 3.2.2.6 and 3.3.3.1.

3.3.4.4 Data access

Access to the Smittestopp backend operates on a component level, with only a handful of people having access to critical components such as Data Lake and SQL Database (notwithstanding the differentiation between the dev and prod environments). All access to customer assets in the Azure subscription were controlled and audited by NHN.

Access by Microsoft: The Data Processing Agreement (DPA) between Microsoft and NHN is the judicial framework that Microsoft depends on with respect to GDPR [11]. According to this agreement, Microsoft is contractually obligated to provide sufficient guarantees to meet key requirements of GDPR.

Access by developers: Access to any services related to data storage and data processing were granted to vetted developers by NHN on a subscription basis. Developer access was granted to a limited number of Simula and NIPH personnel.

3.3.4.5 Bluetooth IDs

A weakness in the first release of Smittestopp was the use of static client IDs for tracing BT pairings. The client ID is exchanged with another instance of Smittestopp when two devices are within BT range of each other. With static IDs, it is possible to non-continuously track users through BT beacons, placed at strategic locations, that scan for the presence of specific IDs. To avoid this type of tracking, the client ID should change over time, which can be achieved by rotating IDs. Therefore, an endpoint (see Section 3.2.2.10) for providing rotating client IDs was implemented, and support for rotating client IDs was added to the mobile app. Using this endpoint, the mobile app can request a set of random client IDs and use each ID for a period before it is changed. When the mobile app runs out of IDs, it requests a new set of

IDs from the backend. This feature was implemented and tested, but never released to the general public.

3.3.4.6 Research and development data

The acquisition of data to use for research and development is often challenging in situations involving personal information. According to the sandbox approach described in Section 3.2, we maintained two instances of the backend system, namely, the dev and prod environments. Here, the prod environment was completely out of reach for the majority of the team, and data collected in the dev database, contributed by the informed volunteers from Simula and NIPH, were available for development purposes. Although this helped us build our algorithms and prototypes, the fact that we were never able to test at the real scale remained a challenge. Nevertheless, this was an important measure to protect the production user data from potentially unstable development versions of the services and functions.

3.4 Summary and conclusions

In this chapter, we presented an overview of the Smittestopp backend solution, elaborating on its purpose, design, implementation, and operations. We traced the evolution of the solution over time as a response to project goals and requirements, reflected upon various aspects of performance, and, finally, touched upon the open challenges that can hopefully motivate future work. The overall Smittestopp system was deployed for public use in only about give weeks, reaching a record 1.5 million registrations in a short time and collecting hundreds of millions of data records. Despite the issues and challenges that still remain to be open, we hope that our experiences and insights can support future projects of a similar nature, by allowing other teams to learn from our mistakes and use our preliminary results.

References

[1] Vilni Verner Holst Bloch (Statistisk Sestralbyrå). Standard for delområde- og grunnkretsinndeling. https://www.ssb.no/klass/klassifikasjoner/ 1(inNorwegian),accessedFebruary2021.
[2] Simula Research Laboratory and Simula Metropolitan. Sammenligning av alternative løsninger for digital smittesporing. https://www.simula. no/sites/default/files/sammenligning_alternative_digital_ smittesporing.pdf(inNorwegian),accessedFebruary2021.
[3] Microsoft. API management. https://azure.microsoft.com/en-us/ services/api-management/,accessedFebruary2021.

[4] Microsoft. Azure IoT Hub documentation. https://docs.microsoft.com/en-us/azure/iot-hub/, accessedFebruary2021.

[5] Microsoft.   Azure   Kubernetes   Service   (AKS).   https://azure.microsoft.com/en-us/services/kubernetes-service/, accessedFebruary2021.

[6] Microsoft.   Azure Maps.   https://azure.microsoft.com/en-us/services/azure-maps/, accessedFebruary2021.

[7] Microsoft.   Azure Monitor.   https://azure.microsoft.com/en-us/services/monitor/, accessedFebruary2021.

[8] Microsoft.   Hyperscale service tier.   https://docs.microsoft.com/en-us/azure/azure-sql/database/service-tier-hyperscale, accessedFebruary2021.

[9] Microsoft.   Introduction   to   Azure   Data   Lake   Storage   Gen2. https://docs.microsoft.com/en-us/azure/storage/blobs/data-lake-storage-introduction, accessedFebruary2021.

[10] Microsoft. Microsoft Azure. https://azure.microsoft.com/en-us/, accessedFebruary2021.

[11] Microsoft. Microsoft's GDPR Commitments to Customers of our Generally Available Enterprise Software Products. https://docs.microsoft.com/en-us/legal/gdpr, accessedFebruary2021.

[12] Microsoft.   Welcome   to   Azure   Stream   Analytics.   https://docs.microsoft.com/en-us/azure/stream-analytics/stream-analytics-introduction, accessedFebruary2021.

[13] Microsoft.   What   is   Azure   Active   Directory   B2C?   https://docs.microsoft.com/en-us/azure/active-directory-b2c/overview, accessedFebruary2021.

[14] Microsoft. What is Azure Data Factory? https://docs.microsoft.com/en-us/azure/data-factory/introduction, accessedFebruary2021.

[15] Helse Norge.   Smittestopp.   https://helsenorge.no/smittestopp, accessedSeptember2020.

[16] norskhelsenett.   Nasjonale e-helseløsninger.   https://www.nhn.no/, accessedFebruary2021.

[17] Helse og omsorgsdepartementet. Forskrift om digital smittesporing og epidemikontroll i anledning utbrudd av Covid-19. https://www.regjeringen.no/contentassets/116076d9a39b473a97d97474048e1fb0/kgl.-res.-27.-mars-digital-smittesporing.pdf(inNorwegian), accessedFebruary2021.

[18] Patrick Howell O'Neill, Tate Ryan-Mosley, and Bobbie Johnson.   A flood of coronavirus apps are tracking us. Now it's time to keep track of them. https://www.technologyreview.com/2020/05/07/1000961/launching-mittr-covid-tracing-tracker, accessedFebruary2021.

[19] OpenStreetMap.   Welcome   to   OpenStreetMap!   https://www.openstreetmap.org/, accessedFebruary2021.

[20] Simula. En ny runde med digital smittesporing? `https://www.simula.no/news/en-ny-runde-med-digital-smittesporing` (inNorwegian), accessedFebruary2021.

[21] Simula. Smittestopp backend. `https://github.com/simula/corona/tree/master/backend/doc` (authorizationrequiredforaccess), accessedFebruary2021.

[22] Wikipedia. COVID-19 apps. `https://en.wikipedia.org/wiki/COVID-19_apps`, accessedFebruary2021.

[23] Wikipedia. Data anonymization. `https://en.wikipedia.org/wiki/Data_anonymization`, accessedFebruary2021.

[24] Wikipedia. Global positioning system. `https://en.wikipedia.org/wiki/Global_Positioning_System`, accessedFebruary2021.

[25] Wikipedia. Google Maps. `https://en.wikipedia.org/wiki/Google_Maps`, accessedFebruary2021.

[26] Wikipedia. Grunnkretser i Norge. `https://no.wikipedia.org/wiki/Grunnkretser_i_Norge`, accessedFebruary2021.

[27] Wikipedia. Haversine formula. `https://en.wikipedia.org/wiki/Haversine_formula`, accessedFebruary2021.

[28] Wikipedia. Nominatim. `https://wiki.openstreetmap.org/wiki/Nominatim`, accessedFebruary2021.

[29] Wikipedia. Overpass API. `https://wiki.openstreetmap.org/wiki/Overpass_API`, accessedFebruary2021.

[30] Wikipedia. Point of interest. `https://en.wikipedia.org/wiki/Point_of_interest`, accessedFebruary2021.

[31] Wikipedia. Pythagorean theorem. `https://en.wikipedia.org/wiki/Pythagorean_theorem`, accessedFebruary2021.

Chapter 4
Smittestopp analytics: Analysis of position data

Vajira Thambawita, Steven A. Hicks, Ewan Jaouen, Pål Halvorsen, and Michael A. Riegler

Abstract Contact tracing applications generally rely on Bluetooth data. This type of data works well to determine whether a contact occurred (smartphones were close to each other) but cannot offer the contextual information GPS data can offer. Did the contact happen on a bus? In a building? And of which type? Are some places recurrent contact locations? By answering such questions, GPS data can help develop more accurate and better-informed contact tracing applications. This chapter describes the ideas and approaches implemented for GPS data within the Smittestopp contact tracing application. We will present the pipeline used and the contribution of GPS data for contextual information, using inferred transport modes and surrounding POIs, showcasing the opportunities in the use of GPS information. Finally, we discuss ethical and privacy considerations, as well as some lessons learned.

V. Thambawita
Department of Holistic Systems, Simula Metropolitan Center for Digital Engineering,
e-mail: vajira@simula.no

S. A. Hicks
Department of Holistic Systems, Simula Metropolitan Center for Digital Engineering,
e-mail: steven@simula.no

E. Jaouen
Department of Machine Intelligence, Simula Metropolitan Center for Digital Engineering,
e-mail: ewan@simula.no

P. Halvorsen
Department of Holistic Systems, Simula Metropolitan Center for Digital Engineering,
Department of Computer Science, Oslo Metropolitan University,
Department of Informatics, University of Oslo
e-mail: paalh@simula.no

M. Riegler
Department of Holistic Systems, Simula Metropolitan Center for Digital Engineering,
Department of Computer Science, UiT The Arctic University of Norway
e-mail: michael@simula.no

A. Elmokashfi et al. (eds.), *Smittestopp – A Case Study on Digital Contact Tracing*,
Simula SpringerBriefs on Computing 11, https://doi.org/10.1007/978-3-031-05466-2_4

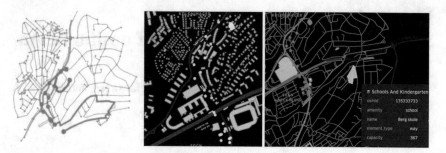

Fig. 4.1: Examples of map prototypes used during the development process. We can see different metadata plotted, such as pathways, buildings, and GPS data points. To create the maps, we used the Kepler library (kepler.gl). Maps created for this pipeline were only used for development and not provided in the final build, due to resource consumption and privacy concerns.

4.1 Introduction

One of the information sources that Smittestopp was supposed to rely on for contact tracing was the position data collected from people's smartphones. Such position data can help determine if people crossed paths and can provide information about the places they visited, such as if someone was in a store or used public transport. Position data, often also referred to as Global Positioning System (GPS) data, usually consist of the position as a longitude and a latitude, as well as a timestamp. Suppose the position data are collected via smartphones. In that case, one can also obtain additional information, such as speed (from one GPS data point to the next), altitude, and accuracy (an approximation of how accurate the obtained position data might be). On the other hand, some GPS data sets contain manually collected data, such as transport modes. For example, the GeoLife GPS Trajectories [11] data set contains annotated trajectories, with labels for the transportation mode (bus, train, walking, and car), latitude, longitude, altitude, and timestamp.

To render raw position data usable for tasks such as contact tracing, pre-processing and pre-analysis are required. First, one needs to extract trajectories from the raw GPS data. These trajectories can be used to find possible intersections and travel paths, among other things. Trajectories and GPS point data are essential for map matching, that is, to connect the GPS information to information obtained from a map. For example, was a person at a bus stop waiting for a bus, was a person in a store, did people walk together, and so on. In addition to map matching and trajectories, identifying a contact also requires analysing which mode of transportation was used (walking, driving, biking, public transportation, etc.) [7]. Moreover, necessary but straightforward pre-processing methods such as bounding box and polygon creation based on GPS points are required. One final challenge that needs to be addressed is that the amount of GPS data is usually massive, with huge numbers of data points (also depending on the granularity of time). Thus, one needs efficient methods to

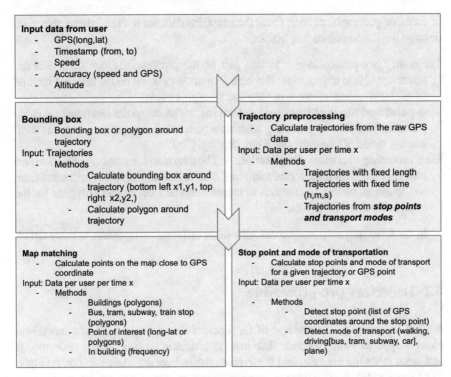

Fig. 4.2: Overview of Smittestopp's GPS analysis pipeline. Raw GPS data are first transformed into trajectories and then combined with metadata from public maps and classified into different transport modes. The processed and enriched data are then used in the contact tracing algorithm.

process the data, especially if nationwide contact tracing is a final goal. Figure 4.1 shows some of the maps used during the development process. The maps contain different types of information, including possible walk paths (left), buildings and GPS data points, (middle), and a more detailed view of certain buildings that shows metadata information such as the name of the school (last).

Based on these general requirements for GPS data analysis, several main objectives arose that needed to be addressed to make the position data useful and usable for the Smittestopp application. These are as follows:

- Trajectory pre-processing.
- Stop point and mode of transport detection.
- Map matching and map visualization.

Figure 4.2 depicts the complete pipeline for the GPS analytics part of Smittestopp. The whole pipeline is implemented in Python and uses different libraries. Details about the libraries used are provided in the respective sections. The pipeline starts with the user data queried from the database. The data can be queried by user, groups of users, or geographical area. Once the raw GPS data are in the pipeline, they pass through the different building blocks.

Trajectory pre-processing: In this part of the pipeline, the raw GPS data are transformed into trajectories. The transformation depends on the selected method (fixed length, time interval, or stop and transport mode).

Stop point and mode of transport detection: The stop point and transport mode part is responsible for detecting whether a person has stopped (e.g. at a bus stop) and the mode of transport (walking, driving, etc.).

Map matching and map visualization: The map matching and visualization part connects the GPS trajectories and point data to meta-information obtained from public maps, including methods to create bounding boxes and polygons for the trajectories for GPS points.

In the following sections, we describe these different components in more detail.

4.2 Trajectory pre-processing

A GPS trajectory is a collection of GPS points describing an object's movement along a specific path. No clear definition is available on how long a trajectory is and what it should contain, and these often depend on the use case. For example, in an application used to track running, different trajectories could be segments of 1 kilometre or specific times, such as a new trajectory every 10 minutes. Another approach could involve a new trajectory for every trip, resulting in a collection of runs. For Smittestopp, we experimented with different ways of creating trajectories from GPS data. The experiments were inspired by related work by [9, 8, 12, 4]. Unlike the related work, we did not have labelled data for our trajectories, so we decided to develop methods that could work unsupervised. The main goal was to keep the methods simple, understandable, and explainable.

From the raw GPS data, we extracted GPS trajectories that could then be used in other analysis steps, such as to find intersections, points of interest (POIs), visited buildings, travel paths, and so forth. Looking at existing systems and the literature, we saw no clear way to extract trajectories that worked the best, but there were different suggestions. For our pipeline, we decided on three different methods:

1. Trajectories with a fixed length of GPS data points.
2. Trajectories with fixed time intervals (hours, minutes, seconds).
3. Trajectories obtained from stop points and transport modes.

The input data for the trajectory pre-processing are GPS data obtained from smartphones per user per time or region. The outputs are the trajectories per user, as a collection of GPS data points.

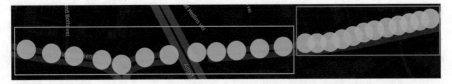

Fig. 4.3: Comparison of changes in a fixed number of GPS points. The green box shows 12 fast-moving GPS points and the red box shows 12 slow-moving GPS points.

4.2.1 Trajectories with a fixed length of GPS data points

In this approach, we divide a long series of GPS data points into trajectories based on a given fixed length. Here, the fixed length is the number of GPS points to be extracted as a single trajectory. Simplicity in handling and processing the trajectories are the main advantages of this method. However, this method's main drawback is that some subtrajectories cover small geographical areas, while others cover large ones. For example, a number N of GPS points for a walking trajectory can be within 1 kilometre, while the same number of GPS points for the trajectory of a fast car can cover around 10 kilometres. To understand this phenomenon, see the illustrations in Figure 4.3. Therefore, when analysing POIs around a trajectory, a large geographical area causes problems in extracting a large amount of additional metadata.

4.2.2 Trajectories with fixed time intervals

In this method, we use predefined time intervals, such as two hours, one hour, half an hour, a minute, and a second to create trajectories. These time intervals are calculated using timestamps, which are part of the metadata of each GPS point collected by the mobile application. The main advantage of this method is its ability to find trajectories for a given time interval. However, similar to the method of extracting a fixed number of points, the resulting trajectories can have an area so large that extracting metadata from the map servers would be too computationally expensive. This function works as a support function to extract POIs from long trajectories, because extracting POIs around a long trajectory is time and resource intensive. The pseudocode of this function is presented in Algorithm 1.

Algorithm 1: Extracting trajectories with fixed time intervals

---

Data: GPSData – A series of GPS points of a trajectory
Result: A list of subtrajectories

timeMode ← SelectTimeMode from (2H, H, HAH, M, S) ;
timeModeInSeconds ← convert timeMode to seconds ;
dividedTimestamp ← GPSdata[timestamp] / timeModeInSeconds ;
uniqueTimestamp ← FindUniqueValues(dividedTimestamp) ;

for $timestamp_i \in uniqueTimestamp$ **do**
    | subTrajectory ← GPSdata[$timestamp == timestamp_i$] ;
    | **Append** $subTrajectory$ to $Result$;
end

4.2.3 Trajectories based on trips and stop points

A natural way of thinking about a trajectory is in terms of different modes of transport. This approach splits a long GPS trajectory into smaller chunk-based trips and stop points. In this case, a trip is defined as moving some distance over some time, such as a person driving to work or walking a dog. Stop points are points where a person is still for a longer period within a predefined radius. The approach is based on the work of Cich et al. [2]. The advantage of this method is that we obtain a clean set of trajectories pertaining to either stop points or trips that can be further classified into a mode of transport. A disadvantage of this method is that we must ensure that the trajectories obtained are stable enough to detect stop points properly and to distinguish between different trips. Furthermore, this method produces trajectories of various lengths. For example, the trajectory of a person going to the post box would be much shorter than that of a person walking to work.

4.3 Predicting the mode of transport

Even if the physical distance between two people is close enough for infection, it does not necessarily mean they were in contact. For example, one person could be driving a car, while the other one is running on the sidewalk. Furthermore, two people can be a safe distance apart but sitting on the same bus, raising the likelihood of infection. Therefore, it was important to assign a mode of transport to the GPS trajectories generated by the users. For this purpose, we defined seven different types of transport modes: being still, walking, running, on a bus, in a car, on a train, and on a plane (see Table 4.1). These categories were selected based on the most common forms of transportation in Oslo, Norway.

Since we were, for the most part, interested in determining whether or not two people were in direct contact with each other, we generalized these groups further to only include *still*, *on foot*, and *in a vehicle* The group *still* covers the case in which a person is standing still, or, in other words, has no speed; *on foot* encompasses all instances of a person moving on foot, such as walking, jogging, or running; and *in a vehicle* contains all cases in which a person is in a vehicle, including seated inside a car, bus, tram, train, or airplane. Despite being a less precise estimation of the transport mode than in using the seven categories above, these categories still achieved our target of being able to more accurately differentiate between in-person contacts. For example, if contact between individuals is determined, but one is *on foot* while the other is *in a vehicle*, we can rule out the possibility of infection. As development continued, we planned to gradually increase the level of precision of the predicted modes of transport, but this was not achieved before the project was shut down.

Research on deriving transport modes from GPS data relies mostly on supervised learning methods that use a large training data set of labelled trajectories to learn the nuances between the different modes of transport automatically (eg, [10, 13, 6, 3]). Since we did not have access to an extensive training data set or time to collect one, we had to settle for a simpler approach using heuristics. We decided to use the speed of a given GPS point to predict its transport mode. This means that we assigned a mode of transport for each point in a given trajectory. Initially, we planned to assign one transport mode per GPS trajectory, but we found that giving each point a transport mode would provide greater flexibility further down the pipeline.

There were two advantages to this method. First, speed was calculated on the smartphones, such that we obtained this information for free, without the need for any additional computations. Second, assigning a transport mode for each point gave us more flexibility in comparing contacts at specific periods of time. The lookup table used to determine transport modes is shown in Table 4.1, where we also show the conjectured speed of the more precise modes of transport. These speed values were selected by taking the average speed of the transport mode in question and adding a small upper buffer to allow for some variability. Since the accuracy of the collected GPS points varied, the assigned transport modes underwent cleaning and post-processing. This involved looking at the individual points within a given time frame and assigning all points within that frame to the majority transport mode.

The evaluation was carried out by comparing the predicted transport modes against a set of manually annotated points collected by members of the development team. Overall, we had approximately 35 test cases for evaluation, all from Simula employees who gave explicit permission to use their data for testing purposes. Each entry consisted of a start time, an end time, and a mode of transport for that duration. The results were evaluated against this test data set continuously through a series of unit tests that ran every time the analytics pipeline was started. Furthermore, we performed a qualitative evaluation of the predicted transport modes using interactive maps generated by kepler.gl.[1] Based on this visual analysis, we made specific changes

---

[1] See https://kepler.gl/.

to the transport mode prediction algorithm, such as the speed thresholds used for the individual transport modes and fixing bugs that were not caught by the unit tests. Despite being very useful in creating a more robust and stable transport mode prediction approach, we had to be careful when making changes, since we were using a small subset of data that might not have represented the overall population. It is important to note that these interactive maps were only used in the development phase of Smittestopp, and not in production.

Mode of Transport	Minimum Speed (km/h)	Maximum Speed (km/h)
Standing Still	-	1
Walking	1	6
Running	6	14
Car | Bus | Tram | Train	14	80
Car | Train	80	150
Train	150	220
Plane	220	-
Standing Still	-	1
Running	1	14
In a Vehicle | Public Transportation	14	-

Table 4.1: The lookup table used to determine the transport modes for a given GPS point. The upper half of the table shows the more precise modes of transport, while the lower half shows the modes of transport used in the final version of Smittestopp.

4.4 Map matching and map visualization

Map matching involves combining GPS data with metadata from publicly available maps. For the Smittestopp project, we tested Google Maps, Azure Maps, and OpenStreetMap[2]. Based on the performance we needed and the amount of metadata available for Norway, we decided to use OpenStreetMap. The methods implemented were partially inspired by other work (a good overview can be found in [1]). Nevertheless, we basically started from scratch, to develop methods specifically designed for contact tracing that could provide the information needed and, at the same time, respect the privacy of users. More details on the OpenStreetMap backend we used to query the information are available in the part describing the backend.

Our goal for the map matching was to understand whether a contact had occurred in a closed environment (e.g. a building or a bus), since this could impact the risk level. Contacts are split into three categories: *inside*, which can be inside a given building or a vehicle or public transportation, *outside*, and *uncertain*, when we lack

---

[2] See https://www.openstreetmap.org.

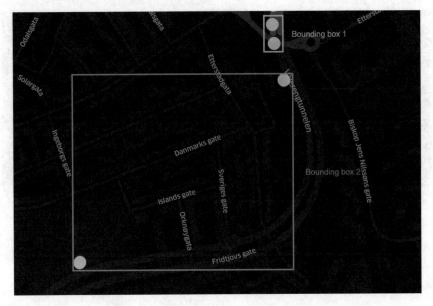

Fig. 4.4: A comparison of two bounding boxes and the areas they cover. Note the differences between the green and red boxes, which both cover the area corresponding to two GPS points.

relevant information or when the data are inconsistent (e.g. one person is detected as being in a car while the other is walking).

4.4.1 Extract POIs from dilated areas

Our main goal is to find POIs around the given trajectories that are associated with positive cases or identified as a trajectory to be analysed. Initially, we considered bounding boxes around trajectories as an area around which to extract POIs. However, the bounding boxes cover a large geographical space than we wanted to analyse to find POIs. The maximum number of unnecessary POI extractions arises when two GPS coordinates are located at two ends of a bounding box's diagonal. Figure 4.4 illustrates this phenomenon. Therefore, we were looking for alternatives, such as extracting POIs using dilated areas.

The main purpose of extracting POIs using a dilated area is to minimize the number of POIs returned for a given trajectory. In this method, we replace the bounding box with a narrowed polygon. The polygon's width (the maximum distance to the polygon boundary from a given point) is defined as an input parameter (a given fixed value). A sample trajectory, a corresponding dilated area, and the extracted POIs within the area are illustrated in Figures 4.5a, 4.5b, and 4.5c, respectively.

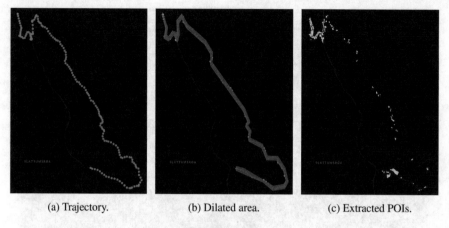

(a) Trajectory.   (b) Dilated area.   (c) Extracted POIs.

Fig. 4.5: An example of a trajectory and its POI extractions using a dilated area.

4.4.2 Obtaining contacted POIs with points

Identifying POIs around a specific GPS coordinate is essential when determining the contacted POIs of a given trajectory. To extract POIs from each GPS point, we consider a circular area around every GPS point of a trajectory, because we did not have access to indoor positioning systems [5]. Practically, when we extract POIs around a point using the radius of a circle, we observe several POIs per point. However, we know that this point could only be in contact with one POI. Therefore, there should be a reliable method to identify the most appropriate POI with a high chance of having contacted a given point.

In this functionality, we can select two options for the value of the radius of the circle, which will be considered the area for extracting POIs. The first option is a fixed radius passed to the algorithm. In this case, we can carry out a heuristic analysis to find the most suitable radius. The second option is to use the accuracy radius, which is part of every GPS coordinate collected by our mobile application. Considering the accuracy value (radius of the accuracy circle) as the radius to extract POIs is logically more related to our goal than the fixed radius, because, when a mobile phone has a poor GPS signal, the radius of the accuracy circle is bigger to extract POIs around it. On the other hand, a large error (when the GPS signal is poor) can lead to a large radius. Then, the POIs cannot be extracted because of there being too much data. To overcome this problem, we defined a threshold for the maximum radius.

Within a single circle, we can sometimes observe several POIs, as mentioned earlier. However, we have to select one of them. We do so by maintaining a ranking score for every POI extracted for a given trajectory. In this scoring method, we increment a counter (starting from zero) when a POI is detected as a contacted POI for a given GPS point. For example, assume that R GPS points intersect with a building B. Then, the rank of building B is R. Ultimately, each and every POI around a given trajectory is assigned a rank based on the number of intersected GPS points. If we detect a single POI for a given point, we consider that POI as contacted. If we have more than one contacted POI, we use the POI with the highest rank. However, if we have numbers of equal rank, we select the first POI detected as the point contacted. The pseudocode for this algorithm is given in Algorithm 2.

Algorithm 2: Obtain the POIs of contacted points.

Data: GPSData, amenities, paddings, maxPadding, columnName,
      OverpassAPI
Result: OutputPerPoint, POIsInfo, POIsCount

GPSOutput ← [ ] ;
POIsInfo ← [ ] ;
POIsCount ← [ ] ;

if *padding is not given* **then**
   | paddings ← List[Minimum(accuracy, maxPadding) for all GPS records];
end

Output ← CallingToOverPassServer(GPSData, amenities, paddings);
OutputPerPoint ← split Output to length of GPSData;
for *POIs in OutputPerPoint* **do**
   | **if** *POIs is not Null* **then**
   | | **append** POIs to POIsInfo;
   | **end**
end

if *POIsInfo is not empty* **then**
   | POIsCount ← CountUniquePOIs(POIsInfo);
end
for *ContactedPOI in POIInfo* **do**
   | ranks ← calculate ranks of ContactedPOI;
   | POIMaxRank ← selectMax(ranks);
   | append POIMaxRank to POIsInfo;
end

4.4.3 Relation between POIs and transport modes

Transport modes and POIs are closely related, since both indicate whether the contact could have happened in a closed environment. We describe this interaction in a few points below.

First, POIs are only queried at instants when the trajectories in contact are associated with transport modes indicating that the contact could indeed have happened. In a nutshell, we will not check whether people considered to be in a car were inside a building. More precisely, we will query POIs for trajectories satisfying the condition that either (i) both are considered to be *on foot* (which covers walking and running) or *still* or (ii) one of the trajectories is considered so and we do not have data for the other (transport mode *N/A*). The result of querying the POIs will lead to their classification as either *outside* or *inside*.

Second, parts of trajectories for which either (i) both are considered inside transport or (ii) one of them is and we lack data for the other will be considered as inside a transport, which means the contact will be classified as *inside*. Table 4.2 summarizes how we first infer the *contact transport modes* from the transport modes of each trajectory. A contact inside transport is considered to occur inside, and looking for POIs will lead to contacts occurring either outside or inside.

Trajectory	Still	On Foot	Public Transport	Vehicle	N/A
Still	Out/Inside	Out/Inside	Uncertain	Uncertain	Out/Inside
On Foot	Out/Inside	Out/Inside	Uncertain	Uncertain	Out/Inside
Public Transport	Uncertain	Uncertain	Inside	Inside	Inside
Vehicle	Uncertain	Uncertain	Inside	Inside	Inside
N/A	Out/Inside	Out/Inside	Inside	Inside	Uncertain

Table 4.2: This table describes how the different contact modes (inside, outside, or uncertain) are informed by the transport modes of the trajectories. For example, if two users who meet have *vehicle* as the transport mode in the same location, the contact is defined as happening inside.

We also apply a smoothing function to the trajectories' transport modes, to detect suspicious transport modes, which involve data we assume to be spurious and due to incorrect transport mode attributions. More precisely, we initially compute whether the different points of the trajectories are those for which we should query POIs or ones judged to be *inside transport*. Afterwards, we smooth this prediction by re-attributing the predicted value for points of contact whose prediction differs from those both before and after. More specifically, we look for points of contact t_i such that contact at t_i is considered inside a vehicle, but contacts at $t_{i-2}, t_{i-1}, t_{i+1}$, and t_{i+2} (where the length of this interval is a parameter) are considered to be walking/still. Such points, if below a certain duration threshold, are transformed into the opposite prediction, which is, in this case, not *inside transport*.

Once this smoothing has been applied to the contact's transport modes, the points are classified as (i) inside a transport (e.g. contact happening inside a car); (ii) points for which people are walking/still and we would like to know if they met outside or, for example, inside a school or a shop; and (iii) points with inconsistent transport modes, whose contact location/context will be considered *uncertain*.

Lastly, the radius of search of POIs depends on the transport mode detected. The reason we generally use a nonzero radius – that is, a point need not strictly be within a polygon, but only very close to it – is to handle GPS imprecision, which can typically be high inside a building. On the other hand, keeping a high radius can lead to trajectories on the pavement being perceived as happening in nearby shops alongside that pavement. A compromise is to first compute a search radius based on the GPS inaccuracy and to apply a coefficient based on the transport mode detected (e.g. equal to 1.0 if both trajectories are *still*, but reduced to half if both are *on foot*).

4.4.4 Querying POIs

Once the transport modes are analysed, the last step of our method to obtain the context of a contact (see *Algorithm 3*) is to query points of interest for parts of the trajectories. First, we feed chunks[3] of these trajectories to the functions mentioned above that query contacted POIs. Second, we apply smoothing to these detected points, very similarly to smoothing we applied to the transport modes. Since we use a nonzero radius to search for POIs, the role of this filtering is to eliminate contact points that actually might not have happened in a closed environment. Such scenarios – isolated trajectory points being attributed to a POI for a short duration – could involve, for example, nearby shops when walking on the pavement.

When querying POIs from OpenStreetMap Overpass, we receive specific information with very precise names[4]. Therefore, we design a dictionary converting the information detected into simple categories names (e.g. we extract the value *dormitory* and convert it into the general term *residential*). We used the following list of (generalized) POIs: hospitals, nursing homes, schools, kindergartens, universities, bars and restaurants, sports facilities, culture and entertainment facilities, residential, religious buildings, shops, other education facilities, other healthcare facilities, and others.

Information returned to reports include the duration of contact within each of the three categories (*inside*, *outside*, and *uncertain*), as well as the types of inside contact (inside a mode of transport or one of the POIs following the aforementioned list) and their respective durations. Moreover, we returned a filtered version of the POIs, keeping only locations above a certain duration and/or relative duration threshold.

The data obtained from the POIs are then part of the information of a given contact. More specifically, the POIs are an attribute of the contacts, and the aforementioned information (duration inside and outside, locations of contacts, transport modes) are stored within dictionaries describing a contact's properties. These dictionaries are used to display results when executing specific code or are sent as JSON objects to the frontend. When producing the reports, one can then retrieve the particular

---

[3] It became progressively clear that, to handle the data we received, we had to compute the nonzero duration of single timestamps. In other words, we interpreted the duration of the segment $[t_i, t_j]$ as roughly $(t_{j+1/2} - t_{i-1/2})$, with $t_{j+1/2}, t_{i-1/2}$ defined using previous and subsequent timestamps. This allows single timestamps to have a nonzero duration. To ensure that we are not capturing excessively long durations (e.g. where the phone stops recording so that $t_{j+1} \gg t_j$), we cut up the trajectories into chunks of typically two hours.

[4] See https://wiki.openstreetmap.org/wiki/Points_of_interest.

locations if contacts between two users occurred, as well as obtain a summarized description of the most important of all the users' contact locations.

4.4.5 Accuracy of the identified POIs

The quality evaluation of the predicted POIs was carried out using data for which we had ground truth generated by members of the Smittestopp development team to test different scenarios and edge cases. Thus, different parts of the code were changed based on these tests (e.g. varying the accuracy with transport modes, asking for one or both individuals to share a specific type of transport mode).

In their definitive form, the POIs seemed accurate and coherent with the ground truth available. However, we have no quantitative figures to more precisely judge their accuracy. Besides, one should bear in mind that several steps filter out potential errors (if they account for a negligible part of the predictions). Such cleaning steps include the generalization of the detected points of entities (a step related to privacy concerns) into more general categories – for example, the algorithm can detect a 'apartment' instead of a 'cabin' and, since both are displayed as being 'residential', the error would be invisible in the reports – as well as the filtering of POIs accounting for a short duration and the relative duration of the contact – for example, if one identifies a 'shop' for a few seconds that was not in the ground truth data, it could be filtered out and again become invisible in the reports.

Algorithm 3: Computing POIs for a contact.

Data: Contact details, incl. locations, timestamps, accuracy. ;
Transport modes of each trajectory.
Result: POIs, duration of contact inside, outside, uncertain.

Get types of transport modes (inside transport, on foot or still, uncertain) for the contact
   from each trajectory's transport modes. ;
Get the radius of search for POIs based on transport modes and accuracy of the contact. ;
Split the contact into chunks of shorter duration (2 hours). ;

for *chunk of trajectory in full trajectory* **do**
   Call 'Get POIs of contacted points' to attribute a POI or none to each trajectory point. ;
   Eliminate 'suspicious PoIs' i.e., indices whose labels are isolated (surrounding
      instants not related to the same POI) and of short duration are filtered out. ;
   Keep only PoIs for which the contact's transport modes are consistent (on foot/still). ;
   Extract building/PoI type and convert it into more general categories.
   for *label type, i.e., some PoI, inside transport, outside, uncertain* **do**
      Get the duration of contact related to that label (e.g. inside transport) by
         computing the duration of consecutive indices of identical label. ;
      Update the total duration of contact inside, outside, uncertain. ;
   end
end

4.5 Challenges, experiences, and lessons learned

The treatment of GPS data led to multiple challenges, as well as being time-consuming and resource intensive. GPS signals often being very imprecise, we had to reconsider early plans to adapt them to typical levels of inaccuracy or issues in the real data gathered. These issues include difficulties in determining transport modes (since successive inaccurate positions can lead to incorrect speed computations) or POIs (forcing us to relax the strict requirement that a point must be within a building's OpenStreetMap polygon to be considered inside it). In addition, we considered leveraging these very difficulties to our advantage, such as attempting to deduce being inside from more inaccurate measurements, which did not perform satisfactorily. Great opportunities are associated with the use of GPS data in combination with external resources such as public maps and metadata, which constitute a powerful tool to infer much information. Many functionalities were eventually left out, not used, or not finished before Smittestopp was shut down, including street map analysis using pathways and distinguishing public transportation use from other personal transportation, among many others. Proper followup studies and more development time would be needed to observe the effects and value of such features for contact tracing.

4.6 Ethical considerations

The use of GPS data raises many questions about data privacy. Since our analysis can trace a person's locations, it allows us to access much personal information. For example, using the collected data, we can determine where a person went to work, when the person left for the gym, and what restaurant the person went to for dinner. Had one kept the raw information from OpenStreetMap, even more sensitive information would have been displayed. We intended to use the minimal amount of informative data, leaving out all that seems unnecessary or ethically questionable. Following that principle, we returned rather general terms (e.g. the residential label instead of an address), protecting more sensitive information (e.g. addresses, names, and the type of apartment a person was visiting). Moreover, one should keep in mind that the personal information mentioned is intrinsic to GPS data, in the sense that we did not add any information sources (e.g. public telephone book entries) that would have allowed for the easy identification of the person, simply using OpenStreetMap, which can be accessed as soon as one acquires GPS data.

To protect privacy, we also exclusively used the data of Simula employees who were part of the Smittestopp application development team and who agreed to being part of the testing. Information from these test subjects and the resulting maps were not made public or shared with anyone besides project management, and then only during the development stage. The data collection and analysis were kept separate. Additionally, later on, we decided to hide sensitive information by not providing the interactive maps created for the development stage in the presentation of the results (since visualizing the movements of users further raised privacy issues), as well as combining relevant information in summary form (e.g. communicating the most common transport modes of a contact, rather than the transport modes for all instances of that contact). No interactive maps were used in the production system, but static maps were implemented within the analysis pipeline.

4.7 Summary and conclusions

We presented and discussed the GPS data analysis pipeline and methods developed for Smittestopp. In addition, we discussed lessons learned and ethical considerations. Overall, we can summarize that GPS data hold a great deal of potential for contact tracing, especially if combined with metadata from public maps and related databases. Nevertheless, this information can be seen as optional and might not be relevant in determining close contacts. This information is also associated with substantial ethical and privacy-related concerns, and one needs to weigh the usefulness and added value against these. For Smittestopp, we implemented the features that we found most useful with the smallest privacy impact, and omitted functionalities such as geomapping/tracking and person identification (which is possible to a certain degree of accuracy with the data at hand, public maps, and the person's registration information).

References

[1] P. Chao, W. Hua, R. Mao, J. Xu, and X. Zhou. A survey and quantitative study on map inference algorithms from gps trajectories. *IEEE Transactions on Knowledge and Data Engineering*, 2020.

[2] G. Cich, L. Knapen, T. Bellemans, D. Janssens, and G. Wets. TRIP/STOP Detection in GPS Traces to Feed Prompted Recall Survey. *Procedia Computer Science*, 52:262 – 269, 2015.

[3] M. Etemad, A. S. Júnior, and S. Matwin. Predicting transportation modes of GPS trajectories using feature engineering and noise removal. *CoRR*, abs/1802.10164, 2018.

[4] R. Mariescu-Istodor, A. Tabarcea, R. Saeidi, and P. Fränti. Low complexity spatial similarity measure of gps trajectories. In *WEBIST (1)*, pages 62–69, 2014.

[5] R. Mautz. Overview of current indoor positioning systems. *Geodezija ir Kartografija*, 35(1):18–22, 2009.

[6] H. Omrani. Predicting travel mode of individuals by machine learning. *Transportation Research Procedia*, 10:840 – 849, 2015. 18th Euro Working Group on Transportation, EWGT 2015, 14-16 July 2015, Delft, The Netherlands.

[7] A. C. Prelipcean, G. Gidófalvi, and Y. O. Susilo. Transportation mode detection – an in-depth review of applicability and reliability. *Transport Reviews*, 37(4):442–464, 2017.

[8] X. Yang, K. Stewart, L. Tang, Z. Xie, and Q. Li. A review of gps trajectories classification based on transportation mode. *Sensors*, 18(11):3741, 2018.

[9] Y. Zheng. Trajectory data mining: an overview. *ACM Transactions on Intelligent Systems and Technology (TIST)*, 6(3):1–41, 2015.

[10] Y. Zheng, Y. Chen, Q. Li, X. Xie, and W.-Y. Ma. Understanding Transportation Based on GPS Data for Web Applications. *ACM Trans. Web*, 4(1), 2010.

[11] Y. Zheng, H. Fu, X. Xie, W.-Y. Ma, and Q. Li. *Geolife GPS trajectory dataset - User Guide*, geolife gps trajectories 1.1 edition, July 2011. Geolife GPS trajectories 1.1.

[12] Y. Zheng, L. Zhang, X. Xie, and W.-Y. Ma. Mining interesting locations and travel sequences from gps trajectories. In *Proceedings of the 18th international conference on World wide web*, pages 791–800, 2009.

[13] F. Zong, Y. Bai, X. Wang, Y. Yuan, and Y. He. Identifying travel mode with GPS data using support vector machines and genetic algorithm. *Information*, 6(2):212–227, 2015.

Chapter 5
Using Bluetooth for contact tracing

Ahmed Elmokashfi and Amund Kvalbein

Abstract Bluetooth data is used as the main method for contact tracing with Smittestopp. When two active devices are within Bluetooth range, they will record the ID of the paired device, along with information about the received signal quality. In this chapter, we describe how this method is implemented in Smittestopp, and how Bluetooth data is processed and analysed, to determine if an encounter between two users should be considered a qualified contact with a risk of contamination. We show that distance estimation based on Bluetooth signals is challenging due to differences between devices, lack of information on transmit power and varying environmental factors. Based on this experience, we propose a simple rule for identifying contacts based on received signal strength combined with information about the operating system type.

5.1 Collecting Bluetooth data from iOS and Android devices

Bluetooth Low Energy (BLE) is a technology for wireless communication in the 2.4 GHz ISM band, and it has been supported by most smartphones since its introduction in 2011 [1]. BLE works over short distances (typically less than 10 metres) and with low capacity (less than 1 Mbps). A BLE device can both advertise its presence by

A. Elmokashfi
Center for Resilient Networks and Applications, Simula Metropolitan Center for Digital Engineering,
e-mail: ahmed@simula.no

A. Kvalbein
Center for Resilient Networks and Applications, Simula Metropolitan Center for Digital Engineering,
Analysys Mason AS,
e-mail: amundk@simula.no

© The Author(s) 2022
A. Elmokashfi et al. (eds.), *Smittestopp − A Case Study on Digital Contact Tracing*,
Simula SpringerBriefs on Computing 11, https://doi.org/10.1007/978-3-031-05466-2_5

broadcasting a unique identifier (Universally Unique Identifier, or UUID) and scan for the presence of a particular UUID in its proximity.

The basic idea for digital contact tracing is to exploit this ability to record when a device with a contact tracing app installed has been in proximity of another device [11]. We refer to such an event as a contact.

A BLE device can assume four different roles that dictate the behaviour of the device: two roles are connection based, while the other two facilitate communication in only one direction. A device assuming a connection-based role can act as a peripheral or a central device. The former is an advertiser, while the latter is a scanner. A central device scans for a particular UUID, connects to it, and can then request extra information. A peripheral device implements a Generic Attribute Profile (GATT) server. GATT defines the way two BLE devices can communicate back and forth using a generic protocol called the Attribute Protocol. Devices following the non-connectable modes act as either broadcasters (i.e. a beacon) or observers (i.e. a scanner), without interaction with other devices. Smittestopp uses connection-based roles, and each device acts as both a peripheral and a central. All devices with the app installed broadcast their UUID and periodically scan for the UUIDs of other Smittestopp devices. Along with the UUID, exchanged BLE packets include information about the transmit power *txPower*. Together with the received power, or received signal strength indicator (RSSI), this information can potentially be used to improve distance estimates. See Chapter 2 for more details. The scan cycles for Android and iOS devices vary:

- Android devices scan for Smittestopp UUIDs every six minutes. If a peripheral is detected, the scan cycle will be reduced to two minutes and will remain so as long as a peripheral is detected. The scan cycle itself lasts about 20 seconds.
- Scanning on iOS devices, however, behaves differently, depending on the state of the app. As explained in Chapter 2, iOS imposes a number of restrictions on BLE exchanges when the app is in the background. An app in the foreground scans continuously for peripherals. Apps in the background, with the screen off, do not scan but can still advertise. Finally, apps in the background while the screen is on scan every five minutes for a period of 10 seconds.

5.2 Challenges in distance estimation using Bluetooth

To detect and classify a contact between two devices, we need an estimate of the distance between them. Smittestopp attempts to estimate this distance based on the measured BLE signal strength at the receiver, denoted the received signal strength (RSS). The RSS is a function of the transmitted power, the gain/loss in the transmitting and receiving antennae, and the signal attenuation (path loss) between the two devices. A simple diagram showing the different components is shown in Figure 5.1.

The radio signal attenuates as the distance between the transmitter and receiver increases. Attenuation can be modelled, and one of the most widely used models is the log distance path loss model [8]:

$$RSS(d) = RSS(d_0) - 10n \log(\frac{d}{d_0}), \qquad (5.1)$$

where $RSS(d)$ (measured in decibel-milliwatt, or dBm) is the signal strength at distance d, $RSS(d_0)$ is the signal strength at the reference distance $d_0 = 1$ metre, and n is an attenuation factor that represents the environment between the two devices. Based on this, the distance can be estimated as follows:

$$d = 10^{\frac{RSS(d_0)-RSS(d)}{10n}}. \qquad (5.2)$$

The BLE standard does not specify the transmit power that should be used by BLE devices. The transmit power level is instead decided by the equipment vendor, within the limits of regulation. The European Standards Organization ETSI allows a maximum transmit power of 10 dBm (20 dBm with adaptive frequency hopping). Some devices allow the transmit power to be adjusted through an application programming interface.

The transmit power is broadcast by the transmitter as part of the beacon advertising packet structure, and is denoted as *txPower*. The advertised *txPower* is meant to indicate $RSS(d_0)$, the received signal power at a distance of 1 metre. For Smittestopp, we use the default transmit power levels for both iOS and Android phones. Android allows the transmit power to be set to *high* or *low*, where the default is low.

There could, however, be a discrepancy between *txPower* and the actual $RSS(d_0)$, due to loss or gain in the transmitter antenna. Similarly, the RSSI recorded at the receiver might not be the actual $RSS(d)$, due to unclear loss/gain in the receiving antenna. These effects will depend on the antenna and make of the terminal equipment. To account for this, several initiatives have been taken to measure the actual $RSS(d_0)$ values for different smartphone models [4, 6]. The goal of these measurements is to calibrate different terminals so that differences can be accounted for when trying to estimate attenuation (as a proxy for distance) based on RSSI values. The current form of Smittestopp does not use such calibrations.

In addition to the uncertainties related to the *txPower* and RSS values, distance estimation is challenging, due to variations in the orientation of transmitters and the environment. It is known that the orientation of a mobile handset can have a significant impact on the measured RSSI. The presence of a human body between

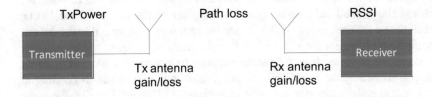

Fig. 5.1: The received signal power is a function of the transmitted power, the gain/loss in transmitting and receiving antennae, and the path loss.

the transmitter and the receiver can reduce the signal strength. Conversely, reflections from walls, ceilings, or floors in an indoor environment can produce a stronger signal than what would be expected from the log distance path loss model. Given these considerations, we do not attempt to use a formula to estimate the distance between two handsets.

5.3 Controlled experiments to aid distance classification

Epidemiologists determine potentially contagious contacts based on the duration two persons were in proximity to each other and the distance between them. As explained above, it is challenging to accurately determine distance based on BLE RSSI measurements. Instead of calculating an exact distance based on each RSSI measurement, Smittestopp classifies a contact as *very close*, *close*, or *relatively close* based on a set of RSSI measurements from a contact. The classification is discussed in Section 5.4. Here, we describe a series of controlled experiments that were carried out to determine suitable thresholds for the classification.

5.3.1 April 2020 signal strength measurements

Several controlled experiments were conducted with a limited set of smartphones in April 2020. Overall, we used 26 phones, 18 of which were iOS and the remainder Android phones, with 10 and eight unique types, respectively (see Table 5.1). These experiments can be broadly split into scenarios in which the phones are kept at a distance of 1 metre (*very close*), 2 metres (*close*), and farther apart (*relatively close*). An overview of the scenarios in each group is given in Table 5.2.

Figure **??** shows the distribution of the RSSI values measured in the different experiments. Experiments with the same operating system (OS) on the transmitter side and distance class are grouped together. We do not distinguish between different OSs on the receiver side. Table 5.3 shows the mean, median, and standard deviation for each class of experiments. First, we observe a clear difference between measurements based on the OS of the transmitting device. The measured signal strength is normally 10–20 dB stronger from iOS devices compared to Android devices. As discussed above, the BLE transmit power is not given by the BLE standard, but is, instead, set by the equipment vendor. These measurements indicate that the default transmit power is higher for iOS devices than for Android devices.

Second, we observe clear differences between measurements taken at different distances. This is good news, since it suggests that it is possible to conduct at least a coarse-grained distance estimation based on RSSI values. For iOS, the mean (median) RSSI is 17.8 dB (21 dB) higher in the experiments in the very close category compared to the close category. For Android, the difference in means (medians) is 10.2 dB (12 dB).

Table 5.1: The phone models that were used in the April 2020 tests.

OS	Phone model	Count
iOS	iPhone 5S	1
iOS	iPhone 6	2
iOS	iPhone 6 Plus	2
iOS	iPhone 7	1
iOS	iPhone 8	1
iOS	iPhone 8 Plus	1
iOS	iPhone X	4
iOS	iPhone XS	2
iOS	iPhone 11 Pro	2
iOS	iPhone 11 Pro Max	2
Android	Xiaomi Mi MIX 2S	1
Android	Samsung Galaxy S5	1
Android	Samsung Galaxy S8	1
Android	Samsung Galaxy S8+	1
Android	Samsung Galaxy S10	1
Android	Google Pixel 3 XL	1
Android	LG Nexus 5	1
Android	Huawei P9	1

Table 5.2: Controlled experiments in April 2020

ID	Transmitting device	Class	Description
1	Android	Very close	Phones 1 metre apart on a table
2	Android	Very close	Phones in same car while driving
3	Android	Very close	Phones on same person while walking/driving
4	Android	Very close	Phones on same person while walking
5	Android	Close	Phones on two persons walking side by side
6	Android	Close	Phones in front/back of car
7	Android	Within range	Phones in adjacent rooms
8	iOS	Very close	Phones 1 metre apart on a table
9	iOS	Very close	Phones in same car while driving
10	iOS	Very close	Phones on same person while walking/driving
11	iOS	Very close	Phones on same person while walking
12	iOS	Close	Phones on two persons walking side by side
13	iOS	Close	Phones on different tables in same room
14	iOS	Within range	Phones in adjacent rooms

Table 5.3: RSSI values for different distances and operating systems

Distance	OS	Mean	Median	Std Dev
Very close	iOS	-54.7 dBm	-51 dBm	17.2 dBm
Very close	Android	-71.8 dBm	-71 dBm	8.4 dBm
Close	iOS	-72.5 dBm	-72 dBm	9.9 dBm
Close	Android	-82.0 dBm	-83 dBm	5.6 dBm

Third, the measurements show a significant variance in the RSSI values. This is particularly true for the iOS very close measurements. This result indicates that the number of samples needed to reliably classify a contact as very close or close can sometimes be significant.

5.3.2 August 2020 extended RSSI experiments

The method for identifying and classifying contacts described in Section 5.4 was developed based on the limited measurements discussed above. To further refine or verify the estimates, we utilize a data set collected in August 2020. These data were collected to assess the efficacy of Smittestopp in detecting contacts. For this purpose, 31 smartphones were spread over a large table, where they continuously gathered RSSI data for three days. The makes and models of these phones were chosen based on the top phones that downloaded Smittestopp. Table 5.4 presents the makes and models of these phones. Figure 5.2 illustrates the physical setup of this experiment. A total of 12 phones (six iOS and six Android phones) had their screen on during the experiment. Of these, six phones (three iOS and three Android phones) had the Smittestopp app running in the foreground.

Figure 5.3 shows the RSSI values gathered from these smartphones. Each pair of smartphones was classified as very close or close, based on the distance between the two phones. A phone is classified as very close if the distance from the receiver is less than 1 metre, and as close otherwise.

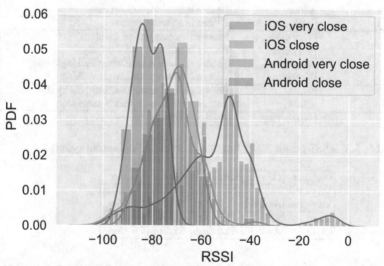

The probability density function (PDF) of RSSI values for different distances and OSs (April 2020)

OS	Phone model	Count
iOS	iPhone 6s	2
iOS	iPhone 8	1
iOS	iPhone XS	2
iOS	iPhone SE	1
iOS	iPhone SE 2nd Gen	5
iOS	iPhone 11 Pro Max	2
iOS	iPhone 11	1
Android	Samsung Galaxy A8	1
Android	Samsung Galaxy A10	1
Android	Samsung Galaxy A50	2
Android	Samsung Galaxy A71	1
Android	Samsung Galaxy S9	1
Android	Samsung Galaxy S9+	1
Android	Samsung Galaxy S10	2
Android	Samsung Galaxy S20 5G	2
Android	Samsung Galaxy Note 10	1
Android	Google Pixel 4	1
Android	LG Nexus 5	1
Android	OnePlus 8	1
Android	Motorola one vision 8	1
Android	Sony Xperia 1	1

Table 5.4: The phone models used in the August 2020 tests.

The results in Figure 5.3 are largely consistent with those of the April measurements in Figure **??**. The same distinction between iOS and Android phones is evident, as is the difference between very close and close phones. The RSSI values measured are, however, higher in the August experiment setup. This can be explained by the smaller (average) distance between the smartphones, given the strict (1-metre) criterion for including a pair of phones in the very close category.

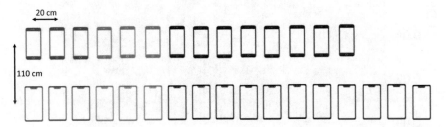

Fig. 5.2: The August measurements were conducted with phones of different makes spread over a table.

5.3.3 The effect of the *txPower* parameter

As discussed in Section 5.2, the *txPower* parameter is included in the messages that are broadcast by the BLE devices. This parameter indicates the expected signal strength at a distance of 1 metre from the transmitter. Figures 5.4 and 5.5 show the distribution of RSSI values for different announced *txPower* values for the iOS very close and Android close groups from the August experiments.

We observe that the *txPower* values vary for both the iOS and Android phones. For the iOS phones, we observe three distinct *txPower* values (from different iPhone models), while we see four distinct values for the Android phones. There are small differences in the RSSI values measured between the different *txPower* values, and it is hard to identify any systematic relation between *txPower* and the RSSI. The results from the April measurements are more dispersed, but they do not provide any basis for systematically concluding that different *txPower* values result in different RSSI observations. Based on these observations, it was decided to not include *txPower* in the contact classification.

As noted above, there were several initiatives to measure the RSS from different phone models in controlled experiments, to compensate for any differences in equipment. The decision to not include *txPower* in the distance estimation process means that we cannot utilize these efforts. This means that there is a risk that we are not adequately capturing differences between the phone models in our contact

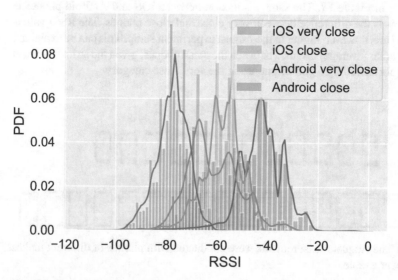

Fig. 5.3: The probability density function (PDF) of RSSI values for different distances and OSs (August 2020)

classification. On the other hand, the *txPower* of different phone models can also be set programmatically, which is not captured by the calibration models.

5.4 Identifying and classifying contacts

There are two main assumptions behind digital contact tracing. First, proximity events that are observed via BLE approximate the underlying physical contact. Second, the BLE signal strength can be used as a reliable proxy for estimating the actual distance between the devices involved. Next, we describe how Smittestopp identifies and describes contacts, along with verification results.

5.4.1 Contact events

An encounter between two mobile phones is a time series of discovery events. Each point in this time series is a tuple of the encounter timestamp and connection properties, which include the measured strength of the signal to the other mobile phone, as well as the other mobile phone's transmission power. In a fully distributed system, each app keeps such a time series locally and uses it later, when identifying

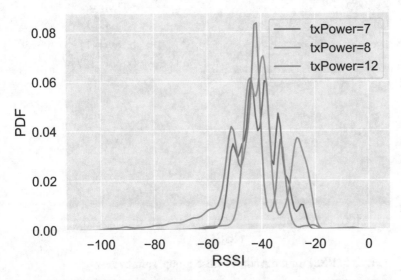

Fig. 5.4: RSSI values for the iOS very close group, split by *txPower*

risky contacts.[1] In a centralized system, such as Smittestopp's, all the time series are uploaded to a central server, for further matching and processing that combine measurements from different phones.

To identify all contacts between two apps A and B within a given time interval $[T_i, T_j]$, Smittestopp follows a two-step approach, which we illustrate in Figure 5.6 and describe as follows:

1. The first step combines the discovery event time series from both devices (i.e. A discovering B, and vice versa) into *contacts*. The combined time series comprise n discovery events $\{e_1, e_2, e_3, ..., e_n\}$, where $n = 5$ in our example.

   Each event e_i is a tuple that consists of four values, $\{ts_i, Ph_1, Ph_2, rssi\}$, where ts_i is the timestamp of the discovery event, Ph_1 is the phone performing the measurement, while Ph_2 is the measured phone. Finally, $rssi$ is the measured signal strength indicator. Smittestopp then considers e_1 as the beginning of a contact and starts looping through the combined discovery time series. Two consecutive events e_i and e_{i+1} belong to the same contact if $ts_{i+1} - ts_i \leq \tau$. Consecutive events spaced by more than τ belong to different contacts. We set τ to five minutes, which allows us to identify contacts, given Smittestopp's scanning rate.

   Recall from Section 5.1 that iOS devices scan every five minutes, while Android devices can take up to six minutes before discovering a nearby device. A contact

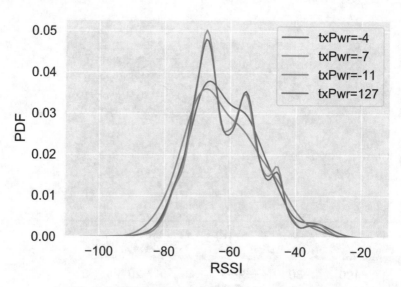

Fig. 5.5: RSSI for the Android close group, split by *txPower*

[1] For an updated list of different contact tracing apps, see https://www.technologyreview.com/2020/05/07/1000961/launching-mittr-covid-tracing-tracker/.

consisting of a single discovery event is assumed to have lasted for five minutes. This results in a time series of contacts $TS_{A,B}$. Each element in this time series is a contact that is characterized by the following: 1) a start timestamp, 2) an end timestamp, and 3) an array of RSSI measurements. Each of these measurements is tagged with the OS of the peripheral. The OS will be used later when determining proximity based on the measured RSSI.

2. BLE scans may not always succeed, due either to iOS limitations when the app is in the background, radio interference and propagation anomalies, or the presence of multiple devices in the app's proximity, which cannot be detected in a single scanning cycle (20 seconds). Hence, Smittestopp leverages its centralized nature to compensate for these artefacts. Smittestopp identifies all devices that both apps A and B have discovered within $[T_i, T_j]$. Assume that there is a third device C that both A and B discovered during the interval of interest. Smittestopp constructs the combined contact time series for A, C and B, C and then overlays these time

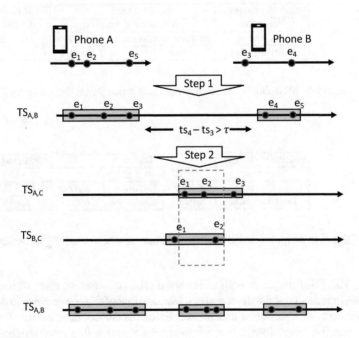

Fig. 5.6: Discovery events from two phones are combined and grouped into contacts.

series over each other to identify all periods where both A discovered C and B discovered C. This results in an intersection time series, $TS_{A,B|C}$, that shows periods when both devices were simultaneously close to a third device. The dashed red rectangle in Figure 5.6 bounds the intersection time series. We refer to this time series extrapolation as *contact graph completion* in the following. Smittestopp next checks whether $TS_{A,B|C}$ includes any contact period that is not in $TS_{A,B}$ and updates the latter accordingly. Note that this update only shows that A and B were close to each other, since both were close to C; it does not, however, include direct RSSI measurements between A and B.

Following the identification of all contact events, Smittestopp maps each event to a single or multiple distance bucket(s) based on the measured RSSI values. The controlled experiments in Section 5.3 shows differences between iOS and Android devices, as well as differences in the measured RSSI values as a function of the distance between phones. Based on these measurements, we define a mapping between RSSI values and the distance categories *very close*, *close*, and *relatively close* as described above. Tables 5.5 and 5.6 present these mappings for the measurements from iOS and Android devices, respectively.

Proximity category	Distance	RSSI range
Very close	$(distance \leq 1metre)$	$(0, -55]$
Close	$1metre < distance \leq 2metres$	$(-55, -65]$
Relatively close	$2metres < distance \leq 5metres$	$(-65, -75]$

Table 5.5: Mapping RSSI to distance categories when detecting an iOS device.

Proximity category	Distance	RSSI range
Very close	$(distance \leq 1metre)$	$(0, -65]$
Close	$1metre < distance \leq 2metres$	$(-65, -75]$
Relatively close	$2metres < distance \leq 5metres$	$(-75, -85]$

Table 5.6: Mapping RSSI to distance buckets when detecting an Android device.

The RSSI ranges in both tables are on the conservative side, which reduces the likelihood of false positives and can increase that of false negatives. To determine the proximity of a particular contact, we divide the contact duration into four proximity ranges (i.e. very close, close, relatively close, and within range), depending on the measured RSSI values. For example, a contact that lasts T_c seconds and involves M RSSI measurements that comprise m_{vc}, m_c, and m_{wr} measurements that fall into the very close, close, and within range buckets, respectively, will be described with the following array, where each element approximates the time spent in each distance bucket: $[(m_{vc}/M)T_c, (m_c/M)T_c, (m_{wr}/M)T_c]$

The contacts that are identified using contact graph completion do not include direct RSSI measurements between the devices of interest. Hence, we leverage the devices' RSSI measurements to a third device to approximate the distance between them. For example, if a is very close to c (i.e. within 1 metre) and b is very close to c, then a and b can be at most 2 metres apart, which corresponds to the case in which c is at the midway point on a straight line between a and b. Generally speaking, the maximum distance between a and b is given by $d(a, b) = max(d(a, c)) + max(d(b, c))$. We use the maximum distance as a conservative measure to classify contact graph completion contacts.

5.4.2 Validation of Smittestopp contacts

To assess the efficacy of Smittestopp in identifying contacts, we use the data set from the experiment with 31 phones, which was described in Section 5.3. This test has similarities to real-world scenarios where a large number of individuals are packed in a limited area, for example, a crowded train or a party, although there are clearly environmental factors in those scenarios that we do capture in this experiment. To this end, we count how many other phones that each phone has seen for at least an hour per day. We choose one hour as a conservative threshold at which Smittestopp will flag a high-risk contact. Perfect identification means that each phone will discover 30 other phones. To quantify the impact of iOS limitations on discoverability, we divide the iPhones in the stress test into three groups: iOS-A, iPhones with the app in the foreground; iOS-B, iPhones with the screen on but the app in background; and iOS-C, iPhones with the screen off.

Figure 5.7 shows the number of phones undiscovered by each test phone during the first test day.[2] The majority of phones discovered 90% of the nearby phones (i.e. 27 other phones). iPhones discovered all the other iPhones, but failed to discover some Android phones. Overall, some Android phones struggled with both discovering other phones, as well as with being discovered. Notably, all Samsung phones exhibited good performance. The three Android phones that struggled the most at discovery were Sony Xperia 1, Google Pixel 4, and OnePlus 8.

Bearing in mind the fundamental limitations of Bluetooth scanning on iOS, we note that Smittestopp performs better than expected on iPhones. Surprisingly, we also observe little difference between the three testing modes for iPhones. A closer look at the Android devices shows that they occasionally suffer from a corrupt Bluetooth cache, which degrades their ability to both scan and be discovered. We believe that this degraded performance is caused by effects unrelated to the app, such as the underlying Bluetooth stack or the way it is managed by Android.

The high level of discoverability can be attributed to the centralized nature of Smittestopp. Figure 5.8 shows that the number of undiscovered contacts doubles and

---

[2] The other two test days exhibit a similar trend.

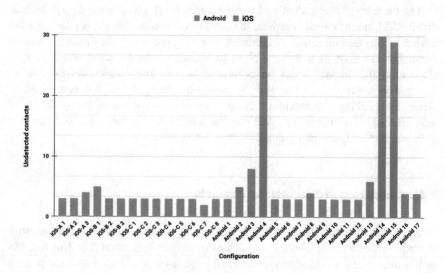

Fig. 5.7: The number of undiscovered phones per test phone on the first test day (iOS-A, iPhones with the app on, in the foreground; iOS-B, iPhones with screen on but with the app in the background; and iOS-C, iPhones with the screen off).

in some cases triples or more when we do not combine time series centrally. As expected, iPhones benefit more from the centralized architecture.

To validate Smittestopp contacts in a realistic setting, we ran a semicontrolled test with participants carrying phones and simulating real-world contacts, such as contacts in training centres, shops, cafes, and public transportation. Overall, Smittestopp performs reasonably well. It correctly identifies 80% of high-risk contacts and is robust to overestimating risk. For more details about the semicontrolled tests and their results, see Chapter 6. For more details about the simulated contacts, see Appendices A and B in [7].

The relatively high accuracy of Smittestopp in both controlled and semicontrolled settings indicates that resorting to RSSI buckets without calibration works acceptably well, with a low number of both false positives and false negatives for high-risk encounters.

5.5 Related work

Since its standardization a decade ago, several works have proposed using BLE for estimating distances indoors (e.g. [10, 18, 13, 9]). These methods assume the deployment of fixed beacons in indoor environments such as shopping centres. Users would then leverage the signal they receive from these beacons to determine their

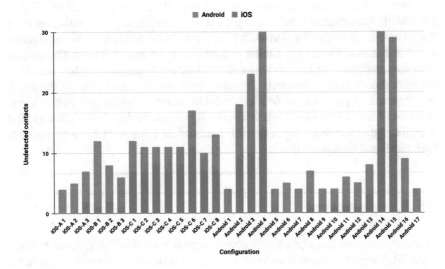

Fig. 5.8: The number of undiscovered phones per test phone on the first test day without *contact graph completion* contacts (iOS-A, iPhones with the app in the foreground; iOS-B, iPhones with the screen on but with the app in the background; iOS-C, iPhones with the screen off).

position. Most previous studies have focused on improving localization accuracy and often report error margins within 2 to 3 metres. Digital contact tracing, however, is different, since it is not built around the presence of fixed beacons, because contacts between people are not limited to indoor environments where such infrastructure can be deployed. Consequently, all involved phones must be both discoverable and be able to discover other devices in their proximity.

The recent interest in using BLE for digital tracing contacts with persons infected with COVID-19 has prompted many to revisit the question of whether BLE can provide an accurate estimate of distance (e.g. [15, 16, 17, 12]). These studies have underscored the difficulty in using BLE RSSI as a reliable estimate of physical distance. Instead, they recommend a set of guidelines (e.g. asking people to put their phones on a table when meeting strangers) or leverage information from other sensors in the phone to determine the context of the contact (i.e. the phone's orientation and placement) to reduce and control for environment-related effects. Notably, the Google/Apple Exposure Notifications (GAEN) framework does not provide a direct mapping between RSSI and distance [5]. Instead, it calibrates phones to control for all device-related effects and then suggests that health authorities determine their own distance thresholds. This task, however, has proved to be harder than expected [3, 14, 7]. Smittestopp opts for using wider ranges to describe contacts, which seems to provide reasonable results.

SwissCovid is one of the contact tracing apps developed based on the GAEN framework. Measurements have been performed to understand the relation between the attenuation reported by SwissCovid and the actual distances between devices [2]. These measurements are similar in nature to those reported here. The goal of the measurements is to find suitable threshold values to determine when identified contacts should lead to an alert. The study presents empirical data on the recall rate (fraction of phones identified within the threshold distance) and precision rate (fraction of identified phones that were actually within the threshold distance). The overall insight from this study is that it is hard to find a threshold that provides both high recall and high precision.

5.6 Lessons learned

In this chapter, we described Smittestopp's approach to identifying contacts using BLE. BLE signal strength is used as a proxy for distance to determine whether a contact between two users is close enough and long enough to warrant notification. In working with BLE contact tracing, we learned, in particular, the importance of the following points:

- The distance should be classified into distance buckets (very close, close, relatively close). A more precise distance estimate seems hardly achievable based on BLE signal strength measurements.
- A higher RSSI sampling frequency can provide more precise estimates. A higher number of RSSI samples will provide greater statistical significance and improve the accuracy of contact tracing. A high sampling rate must be weighed against the added power drain from the device.
- We believe that contextual information about the measurement situation can help guide distance estimation or classification. Such contextual information can include whether the phone is still or moving, whether it is held to the ear or in a pocket, and so forth.
- BLE signal strength can be an unreliable proxy of distance. Still, the simple approach that Smittestopp follows has yielded reasonably good results in both controlled and real-life scenarios.

We believe that all solutions that adopt BLE for contact tracing will need to continuously monitor and improve the mapping between the measured signal strength and proximity. One such improvement could be to use other sensors in the phone to provide extra data to improve BLE localization.

References

[1] Specification of the Bluetooth System, Covered Core Package, Version: 4.0;

The Bluetooth Special Interest Group: Kirkland, WA, USA, 2010.

[2] Swisscovid exposure score calculation, note = "https://github.com/admin-ch/PT-System-Documents/blob/master/SwissCovid-ExposureScore.pdf", year = 2020.

[3] "https://www.thelocal.dk/20200924/what-you-need-to-know-about-technical-error-with-denmarks-smittestop-covid-19-app", year = 2020.

[4] Exposure Notifications BLE calibration calculation , 2020. https://developers.google.com/android/exposure-notifications/ble-attenuation-computation.

[5] GAEN, 2020. "https://covid19.apple.com/contacttracing".

[6] opentrace-calibration , 2020. https://github.com/opentrace-community/opentrace-calibration/blob/master/Trial\%20Methodologies.md.

[7] Sammenligning av alternative løsninger for digital smittesporing, Simula Research Laboratory, 2020. https://www.simula.no/sites/default/files/sammenligning_alternative_digital_smittesporing.pdf, 2020.

[8] J. B. Andersen, T. S. Rappaport, and S. Yoshida. Propagation measurements and models for wireless communications channels. *IEEE Communications Magazine*, 33(1):42–49, 1995.

[9] P. Dickinson, G. Cielniak, O. Szymanezyk, and M. Mannion. Indoor positioning of shoppers using a network of bluetooth low energy beacons. In *2016 International Conference on Indoor Positioning and Indoor Navigation (IPIN)*, pages 1–8. IEEE, 2016.

[10] R. Faragher and R. Harle. Location fingerprinting with Bluetooth low energy beacons. *IEEE journal on Selected Areas in Communications*, 33(11):2418–2428, 2015.

[11] L. Ferretti, C. Wymant, M. Kendall, L. Zhao, A. Nurtay, L. Abeler-Dörner, M. Parker, D. Bonsall, and C. Fraser. Quantifying SARS-CoV-2 transmission suggests epidemic control with digital contact tracing. *Science*, 368(6491), 2020.

[12] G. F. Hatke, M. Montanari, S. Appadwedula, M. Wentz, J. Meklenburg, L. Ivers, J. Watson, and P. Fiore. Using Bluetooth Low Energy (BLE) signal strength estimation to facilitate contact tracing for COVID-19. *arXiv preprint arXiv:2006.15711*, 2020.

[13] P. Kriz, F. Maly, and T. Kozel. Improving indoor localization using bluetooth low energy beacons. *Mobile Information Systems*, 2016, 2016.

[14] D. Leith and S. Farrell. GAEN Due Diligence: Verifying The Google/Apple Covid Exposure Notification API. *CoronaDef21, Proceedings of NDSS '21*, 2021, 2020.

[15] D. J. Leith and S. Farrell. Coronavirus Contact Tracing: Evaluating The Potential Of Using Bluetooth Received Signal Strength For Proximity Detection. 2020.

[16] D. J. Leith and S. Farrell. Measurement-based evaluation of google/apple exposure notification api for proximity detection in a commuter bus. *arXiv preprint arXiv:2006.08543*, 2020.

[17] D. J. Leith and S. Farrell. Measurement-based evaluation of Google/Apple Exposure Notification API for proximity detection in a light-rail tram. *PloS one*, 15(9):e0239943, 2020.

[18] Y. Zhuang, J. Yang, Y. Li, L. Qi, and N. El-Sheimy. Smartphone-based indoor localization with bluetooth low energy beacons. *Sensors*, 16(5):596, 2016.

Chapter 6
Digital tracing, validation, and reporting

Ahmed Elmokashfi, Simon Funke, Timo Klock, Miroslav Kuchta, Valeriya Naumova, and Julie Uv

Abstract Manual contact tracing has been a key component in controlling the outbreak of the COVID-19 pandemic. The identification and isolation of close contacts of confirmed cases have successfully interrupted transmission chains and reduced the disease spread. Even though manual contact tracing has been widely used, its practice has shown that it is slow and cannot be scaled up once the epidemic grows beyond the early phase. In this case, digital contact tracing can play a significant role in controlling the pandemic. In this chapter, based on our experience and lessons learned from the Smittestopp project, we discuss the main prerequisites for the efficient implementation and validation of digital contact tracing in a population. Specifically, we discuss how to translate a close contact defined for manual tracing to proximity events discovered by a phone, that is, how to define a meaningful risk

A. Elmokashfi
Center for Resilient Networks and Applications, Simula Metropolitan Center for Digital Engineering,
e-mail: ahmed@simula.no

S. Funke
Department of Numerical Analysis and Scientific Computing, Simula Research Laboratory
e-mail: simon@simula.no

T. Klock
Department of Numerical Analysis and Scientific Computing, Simula Research Laboratory
e-mail: timo@simula.no

M. Kuchta
Department of Numerical Analysis and Scientific Computing, Simula Research Laboratory
e-mail: miroslav@simula.no

V. Naumova
Department of Machine Intelligence, Simula Metropolitan Center for Digital Engineering,
Simula Consulting AS, e-mail: valeriya@simula.no

J. Uv
Department of Computational Physiology, Simula Research Laboratory
e-mail: julie@simula.no

score and validate the digital contact tracing. We discuss challenges related to each step and provide solutions to some of them, even though questions still remain.

6.1 Manual versus digital Tracing

Since the beginning of the COVID-19 outbreak, contact tracing has been a key component of response strategies in many countries. The rapid identification and quarantine of close contacts of confirmed cases have successfully interrupted transmission chains and reduced the spread of the disease. At the same time, manual contact tracing is slow and cannot be scaled up once the epidemic grows beyond the early phase. Some confirmed cases can also have hundreds of close contacts, as has been reported in the news. To identify, find, and inform all of them in a short time requires a lot of human resources and tedious manual work.

Ferretti et al. propose that digital contact tracing can play a significant role in the control of the COVID-19 pandemic [6]. Since then, several countries have pursued digital solutions for contact tracing using mobile phones. The central idea for digital contact tracing is that individuals in a population install an app that recalls proximity events with other similarly equipped users and then notifies past contacts if and when the individual tests positive for COVID-19. Digital contact tracing does not intend to substitute for manual contact tracing; rather, it allows for the faster and more efficient identification/isolation of close contacts. In this chapter, we discuss how one can correctly identify the most relevant contact events with a digital contact tracing tool and under what circumstances digital contact tracing can be beneficial, compared to manual contact tracing.

The overarching issue we aim to resolve here is how to map proximity events between phones and convert them to epidemiologically meaningful levels of infection transmission risk. To address this issue, we collaborated closely with epidemiologists and manual contact tracing teams from the Norwegian National Institute of Public Health (NIPH). Specifically, we studied the following questions:

- How can one translate a definition of a close contact to proximity events discovered by a phone?
- What is a meaningful definition of a risk score to rank proximity events and contacts?
- How can one validate the digital tracing technology in a population?
- What are the strengths and weaknesses of digital tracing compared to manual tracing?

Manual contact tracing. According to NIPH, close contacts are all people who have been in close contact with an individual who tested positive for COVID-19 in the 48 hours before symptom onset and until that individual comes out of isolation. A distinction is made between 'household members and equivalent close contacts' and 'other close contacts'. The person responsible for contact tracing decides in which category the individual belongs after assessing the infection risk. The type of followup required, including the duration of quarantine, differs depending on the type of contact.

'Household members or equivalent close contacts' are those who live in the same household, those who have had a similar close contact as someone in a household (e.g. boyfriend/girlfriend, work colleagues in an open plan office, the same cohort at a childcare centre or school), and those who have cared for a person confirmed to have COVID-19 without using the recommended protective equipment. Other close contacts are defined as follows

- Any person closer than 2 metres for more than 15 minutes continuously indoors.
- Any person closer than 2 metres for more than 15 minutes continuously, face to face, outdoors.
- Any person who has been in direct physical contact (e.g. shaken hands).

Smittestopp as a digital contact tracing tool. The Smittestopp app was launched on 16 April 2020 with two main objectives in mind:

1. To rapidly alert users by SMS if they have been in close contact with another app user who was later confirmed to have COVID-19.
2. To use the anonymized data collected through Smittestopp and stored centrally to measure the extent to which people are maintaining their distance from each other at the population level, particularly as control measures are gradually relaxed (see Chapter 7).

Smittestopp uses both GPS positioning and Bluetooth (BT) proximity to identify close contacts of confirmed COVID-19 cases. Data are stored for a maximum of 30 days.

For the purpose of contact tracing, Smittestopp has been linked with the Norwegian Surveillance System for Communicable Diseases (MSIS). Since COVID-19 is a notifiable condition in Norway, all laboratory-confirmed cases are registered in the MSIS database, which is required under the regulations on the notification system for communicable diseases. Cases are registered in the MSIS database using the infected individual's national identity number, a unique identifier that is assigned to each citizen or legal resident for life. This record can then be linked to a Smittestopp user's mobile number, which is available through the central Contact and Reservation Register. Only people who have downloaded the app and accepted the terms of use will have MSIS case information linked to mobile contact information. If a Smittestopp user tests positive for COVID-19, other Smittestopp users can be alerted if they were in close contact with that individual in the past seven days before the test.

In Smittestopp, BT data are primarily used to determine proximity between phones, whereas GPS data allow for the identification of locations and the more accurate identification of contact duration. The adapted digital definition of a contact is any person in contact with a case with cumulative BT proximity for more than 15 minutes or at least one instance of BT proximity (i.e. that corresponds to a duration of up to five minutes) and GPS proximity for at least 30 minutes. This definition allows us to identify potential close contacts who were in proximity for less than 15 minutes continuously but, for instance, multiple times over the past days, such as when taking the same bus. At the same time, these types of contacts are completely unnoticed or ignored in the current definition of manual tracing.

After identifying close contacts, the app associates each contact with a risk score/category that helps separate out contacts likely to have resulted in an infection. This scoring is necessary for reducing false alarms, which can potentially lead to requesting healthy individuals to quarantine, or vice versa. The risk score, which has been adapted from the literature and discussions with UK collaborators, is calculated as

$$\int_0^T \frac{1}{\text{distance}^2} dt,$$

where T denotes the accumulated contact time [6, 8]. The inverse distance squared is used to model the spread of droplets generated by coughing [4]. The formula also indicates that the risk is high within 1 metre, where such proximity is expected to be related to physical contact between individuals. The time component helps in weighting the risk; that is, the longer the contact time, the higher the risk.

Another important aspect of risk scoring is the time difference between the contact event and symptom onset. This measure is not captured directly in the risk score, but, rather, implicitly when choosing persons to alert. Recall that Smittestopp only alerts app users who were in close proximity to an infected user in the seven days leading to the test day. The number of days (seven) is treated as a parameter and can be adjusted based on new knowledge related to the disease spread.

The risk scores are calculated separately for BT and GPS contacts. Once these risk scores are calculated, a risk category (low, medium, or high) is assigned to each contact. If BT and GPS contacts result in different risk categories, the highest level of risk is chosen as the ultimate risk category.

	Low	Medium	High
BT data	>15 min	>25 min	>40 min
GPS data	>30 min	>60 min	>90 min

Table 6.1: Correspondence between risk categories and duration of contact at a distance of 2 metres for BT data and a distance of 4 metres for GPS data.

Challenges related to digital contact tracing. From the early phase of the Smittestopp development, we used different approaches to calibrate and validate Smittestopp as a contact tracing tool. These include pre-launch technical validation, comparison of manual and digital tracing in municipalities, and testing in controlled real-life and lab scenarios (see Section 6.4).

During these efforts, it became clear that the definition of digital close contact and risk scores had to be thoroughly tested, adjusted, and validated, due to several factors. This was also pointed out in [6, 10]. First, digital tracing is generally a completely new technology, developed within an extremely short period. Therefore, it still continues to lack technical and epidemiological validation and proper interpretation of the obtained information. Specifically, as pointed out in several studies, the use of neither BT nor GPS signals for digital contact tracing can be expected to deliver optimal results in terms of specificity and sensitivity. For example, as also discussed in previous chapters, the accuracy of a GPS signal is quite low (at least 5 metres), which, by default, does not allow for close contact identification. Even though the BT technology allows us to identify phones in close proximity, the strength of the BT signal changes drastically from one phone to another, as well as based on the phone's location, such as held in a hand or in a pocket. Therefore, it is almost impossible (and not recommended) to translate BT signal strength into the distance definition that is used as input for risk score calculation.

Second, real-life validation of digital contact tracing is particularly challenging, unless a large number of users in a population installs the app (see Chapter 7). In addition, once the contacts of an infected person are identified, how can we ensure that our risk score allows their ranking so that we can notify those who are or will become infected (to notify and quarantine true positives), avoid failing to notify those who are or will become sick (to avoid missing false negatives), and avoid notifying those who are not and will not become sick (to avoid quarantining false positives)? No system will be perfect, and it is important to find the optimal trade-off between these outcomes in terms of the best possible control of the epidemic while still ensuring trust in the technology.

In this chapter, we aim to answer some of the questions, discuss related challenges, as well as share the lessons learned. The chapter is organised as follows. In Section 6.2, we discuss what type of information can be provided by a digital contact tracing tool for its validation and to justify its usefulness for epidemiologists and manual contact tracing teams. Section 6.3 discusses how this information can be obtained from the digital tracing app. In Section 6.4, we discuss the testing and validation routines used for the Smittestopp app, together with the relevant results. We conclude the chapter with a discussion in Section 6.5.

6.2 The type of information necessary to validate a digital tracing tool and prove its usefulness for epidemiologists/researchers

The information generated by the Smittestopp tracing tool is used in three scenarios: first, for the internal validation of the tracing algorithms; second, to support epidemiologists in the contact tracing of infected individuals; and third, to provide aggregated contact and movement statistics at the population level to help decision makers understand the risk of future outbreaks. During the development of Smittestopp, many discussions took place between epidemiologists, researchers, and developers to identify the type of information a tracing tool should provide to tackle these objectives. This sections summarizes the main conclusions for the first two objectives. For the last objective, we refer the reader to Chapter 7.

The key information required to aid in contact tracing is the list of persons who have been in contact with an infected individual. For each person, the system must provide the details, such as the phone number, times, distances, and duration, of the contact with the infected individual. In addition, it is common to present a risk category that summarizes the overall risk of infection transmission in a simple traffic light system (low/medium/high). The risk category allows for the rapid separation between high-risk contacts, which might need immediate action, and medium-risk contacts, which should be looked at in more detail. At times, there can be a high number of contacts, making it necessary to appropriately filter out events we do not consider to be contacts, such as contact involving short durations and/or large distances. In these cases, a risk category provides a natural value for filtering out nonsignificant events. In addition to this key information, the contact's location data can serve as a helpful tool. For instance, knowing if the contact happened inside (within a closed environment) or outside and further being able to determine the type of location – for example, a shop, a public transportation vehicle, or a gym – can help epidemiologists better judge the true risk level of the affected parties. Finally, we found that most of the data can be summarized on a daily basis to obtain a trade-off between sufficient information and compact presentation of the data.

The purpose of internal validation is to evaluate the performance and accuracy of the tracing app, as well as to identify weaknesses. Once a weakness has been identified, it can be addressed and the performance of the tracing increased (e.g. through parameter tweaking or adapted algorithms). To enable the internal validation of the tracing algorithms, the platform must therefore provide sufficient information about contacts, such that they can be compared to reference data. This information can be at a more detailed level than necessary for epidemiologists. For instance, all contact events could be shown, instead of daily aggregated data. The data collection for the internal validation was carried out through pre-launch testing as described in Section 6.4. From this pre-launch testing, we were able to check if the algorithm could correctly identify when the contact happened, the duration of contact, and the location and activity and their durations. The location and activity and their durations were investigated using points of interest and transport modes.

6.3   Obtaining the information: Design principles and the implementation of digital contact tracing

The workflow of the Smittestopp contact tracing pipeline mimics that of manual contact tracing. This means that input to the pipeline involves a time window of interest and a specific individual identifiable via the individual's UUID, and the output is a report summarizing the contact details with other individuals in the population. An important security aspect is that working with the pipeline does not require direct access to the central data storage, because the required data are automatically queried as part of the contact tracing pipeline. In addition, the analysis

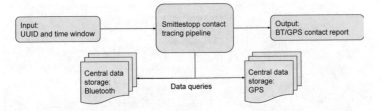

Fig. 6.1: The input to the Smittestopp contact tracing pipeline is a potentially infected individual (identified by a Universally Unique Identifier, or UUID) and a time window of interest. The pipeline returns a report summarizing all BT and/or GPS contacts with other individuals in the population. This process thus mimics manual contact tracing as performed by health authorities. The central data storage can only be accessed from within the automated contact tracing pipeline through a set of predefined queries, thus preventing access to the data outside of contact tracing requests.

pipeline code has only limited access to the GPS and BT data, through predefined database queries. The basic workflow is detailed in Figure 6.1.

In this section, we focus on describing the contact tracing pipeline, that is, the component in the middle of Figure 6.1. The first part details implementation aspects that are shared for processing and analysing both BT and GPS data. However, since the data sources naturally differ and different types of pre-processing are required, the second and third parts describe additional details for GPS and BT data, respectively. The final part then concerns the output of the pipeline, that is, the contact reports.

6.3.1 Shared components between GPS and BT data

Whether we work with BT or GPS data, the main data structure behind the contact tracing pipeline is a contact graph whose nodes represent individuals and the edges between two nodes indicate contacts between the corresponding individuals. Hypothetically, it is possible to constantly maintain an updated version of such a graph over the entire population and for a given time window, but such a strategy is not scalable to reasonable population sizes (larger than a few thousand) and is therefore not pursued. Instead, we compute, on demand, the subgraph of first-order neighbours linked to a potentially infected individual and generate the contact report from the corresponding subgraph. Guided by the number of quarantine days in Norway after potential infection with the coronavirus, the edges in the graph are deleted after 10 days without a contact between two respective individuals. Whenever we refer to the contact graph from now on, we mean the subgraph consisting of the first-order neighbours linked to the input individual.

We note that, at the cost of higher computational demand, the approach can naturally be extended to trace higher-order contacts of a potentially infected individual

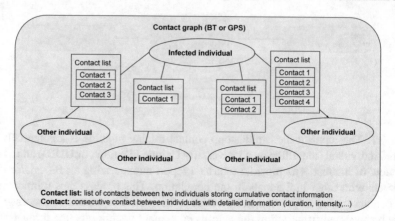

Fig. 6.2: The data structure behind the Smittestopp contact tracing pipeline, which is fed into the summary report generating code. A contact graph is created for each infected individual (with the input UUID) and other users in the central data storage. The edges of the graph contain contact list objects that store all cumulative and detailed information about contacts between two individuals in the time window of interest.

by computing a larger subgraph of higher-order neighbours. To facilitate quick and efficient contact tracing, however, the entire process of on-demand report generation should be facilitated to complete in less than an hour, using limited computational resources. This is because digital contact tracing is most important in times of high infection loads, when hundreds or thousands of pipeline requests can be submitted each day. Furthermore, multiple requests can naturally be run in parallel, so that the parallelization of a single request would require large amounts of overall computational resources.

The core of the codebase consists of three classes that represent contact graphs, contacts, and so-called contact lists (see Figure 6.2). The nodes in the contact graph represent individuals, and the edges of the graph contain instantiations of the contact list class. The contact list object is a list of isolated contacts between the same two individuals that occurred over the entire time window. The representation of contacts using isolated contact events and accumulated contact lists is convenient for report generation, because we can attribute detailed information about each isolated contact event (duration, intensity, location, and more) to instantiations of the contact class, whereas contact list objects can be used to compute cumulative information about all contacts between two individuals in the time window of interest. We note, however, that the noisy nature of both GPS and BT data often fragments an isolated contact between individuals into several contact events, for example, due to loss of BT connection or GPS information, even though all segments belong to the same consecutive contact event. We therefore use merging and interpolation procedures to post-process contact events before deciding whether computed contact events constitute two separate entries in a contact list or should be combined into a single entry by interpolating events. Since the processes of interpolation and merging differ between BT and GPS data, we postpone further details to Sections 6.3.2 and 6.3.3, respectively.

Generating the populated data structure in Figure 6.2 requires the computation of isolated contact events based on information in the central data storage. Due to the different nature of stored BT and GPS data, however, we face vastly different challenges in contact computations based on the data type. We therefore postpone the details of this issue to the next two sections.

Finally, contact summary report generation using a populated contact graph is straightforward, because we can loop over edges to list contacts between two individuals with as much information as we desire. Furthermore, it is only at this point that we filter out certain contacts or individuals based on requirements that are specified by epidemiologists. For instance, we can check whether the cumulative contact list contains contacts with a distance of less than 2 metres over at least 15 minutes and thus report only those contacts satisfying the given specifications.

6.3.2 BT data processing

Querying the central data storage of BT data with a patient UUID and a time window results in a table of events, where each event is specified by the time coordinates (beginning and end) and identifiers of the two devices in contact. In addition, based on the physical proximity, d, of the devices, each event carries information about the duration of very close ($d \leq 2m$), close ($2m < d \leq 5m$), and relatively close ($5m < d \leq 15m$) contacts, which are relevant for determining the risk category (see Table 6.2).

From the point of view of Section 6.3.1, a BT contact graph is straightforward to instantiate, since the nodes and edges are readily available from the query result. However, computing the elements of the contact list require pre-processing, which takes into account the nature of BT event reporting, for example, fragmentation.

Figure 6.3 shows examples of the three scenarios commonly encountered in the BT records: (i) a new BT event occurs entirely within the lifetime of a different event, (ii) two events occur in close[1] succession, and (iii) the events overlap. In such cases, it is not desirable to report the individual BT events as separate contacts (i.e. as different items in the contact list), since this can lead to incorrect (overestimated) risk scores. Instead, items (i) to (iii) are *merged* into a new event to be reported as a contact. The closeness attributes of the new contact, in items (i) and (ii), are computed conservatively, that is, by taking the maximum values of the parent attributes. In the case of overlap, the duration q_C of the child event is computed as

$$q_C = q_A \frac{\Delta_A - \Delta}{\Delta_A} + q_B \frac{\Delta_B - \Delta}{\Delta_B} + \max\left(\frac{q_A}{\Delta_A}, \frac{q_B}{\Delta_B}\right)\Delta,$$

---

[1] The temporal distance of BT events to be considered close is a parameter of the analysis pipeline (see δt in Figure 6.3).

where q_i, Δ_i, $i = A, B$, are, respectively, the attribute values and durations of the parent events, and Δ is the size of the overlap. We remark that the merge rules (i) to (iii) are applied to the list of BT events until no more merging criteria are met (see Figure 6.3 for illustration).

If the GPS data are available, the final step of BT pre-processing is the query of GPS coordinates for each of the contacts in the contact list. The BT events can thus be anchored in space, which is useful, for example, for visualization.

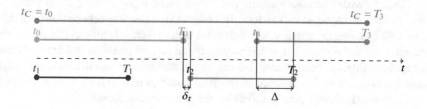

Fig. 6.3: Merging of BT events. Event 0 (lasting from t_0 to T_0, with duration $\Delta_0 = T_0 - t_0$) contains event 1 and is close to event 2 ($t_2 - T_0 \leq \delta_t$). Event 2 overlaps with event 3 for a time $\Delta = T_2 - t_3$. Applying the merge rules to events 0, 1, 2, and 3 results in the final BT contact $[t_c, T_C]$.

6.3.3 GPS data processing

GPS data serve two main purposes when performing digital contract tracing: 1) extracting metadata, such as trajectory maps, to provide a context for a contact, and 2) identifying people who have been in contact with a confirmed case, by computing all GPS trajectories that intersect, for example, for at least 30 minutes with the GPS trajectory of the case. For both these tasks, the raw GPS data are too noisy and require pre-processing, such as removing outliers and, potentially, interpolation.

The algorithm for computing all trajectory intersections must be carefully designed to be computationally feasible. In particular, querying the location data of all other users to check for possible contacts can be costly, due to the size of the data, namely, billions of GPS data points collected within a day. We note that the related queries can be greatly accelerated if the underlying database uses spatial indexing, implemented, for example, as B-trees [2] or R-trees [7]. In particular, collisions can be quickly computed using a hierarchy of bounding boxes (see Figure 6.5 for illustration). While the SQL server used by the Smittestopp backend supports spatial indexing, this solution was not pursued for two reasons: first, the native implementation requires two-dimensional spatial data, and, in our case, the spatiotemporal coordinates are three dimensional. Second, in the centralized database, the depth of the search tree to obtain leaf-node boxes of small volume is considerable. At the same time, a shallow structure means that, at the finest level, ~ 10 square kilometres are searched for contacts.

In the absence of database spatial indexing, the contacts are instead computed in the following hierarchical way. First, on a coarse level, potential contacts are identified through database queries that can be executed quickly on the data storage side. Second, on a fine level, we confir each potential contact by comparing pairs of GPS trajectories. Our intersection algorithm consists of the following steps:

1. The GPS trajectory of the infected case for the analysis period is queried from the database, using a single SQL statement.
2. A list of potential intersection trajectories is computed, using coarse-level contact computation using bounding boxes. The main idea of the algorithm is to

   a. Overlay the trajectory of the case with a minimal set of bounding boxes. The bounding boxes are constructed so that they all have roughly the same volume. Special cases are treated, for instance, if a person travels too fast, as in an airplane.
   b. Query the database for all GPS events within that bounding box. This query is fast because database indices are used for all query parameters, that is, the latitude, longitude, and timestamp.

   The algorithm is visualized in Figure 6.4.
3. All potential intersection trajectories are tested if they have a real intersection with the case trajectory, by computing the distance between all trajectory pairs. For each trajectory pair, the distance is computed for the following methods:

   a. Linear interpolation of the trajectories on the union of their timestamps;
   b. Splitting the trajectories into consecutive segments with no large gaps in either time or space;
   c. Comparing the trajectories on each segment to determine whether a contact has occurred, that is, if the distance is below the predefined threshold.

Figure 6.6 shows an example of the output of this algorithm.

We note that Step 3 of the intersection algorithm described is rather nontrivial, due to the imperfect nature of GPS data and frequent losses of GPS signals (for a recent study of accuracy in urban areas, see, e.g. [12]). First, interpolating GPS data onto the union of the timestamps of both trajectories must not be performed over large gaps in either the spatial or time domain, because this quickly becomes an extrapolation of data, rather than an interpolation. In the Smittestopp contact tracing pipeline, we therefore introduce two parameters specifying the maximum allowed time interpolation (with a default of one hour) and spatial interpolation (with a default of 1 kilometre). Second, even though the GPS data recorded by mobile phones are processed and assisted by data from cellular base stations (assisted GPS [5]), the data still contain extreme outliers that should not be used as valid location points. Fortunately, because of the internal processing of GPS data, mobile phones also return an accuracy measurement with each data point, so that we can exclude extreme outliers by omitting data whose accuracy exceeds a predefined threshold (instances with a default of 50 metres). To facilitate both of these processing tasks, it

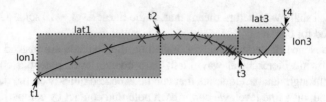

Fig. 6.4: Coarse-scale algorithm for finding all GPS trajectories that intersect with the trajectory of a patient. The patient's trajectory, represented by the black line with a red cross indicating the position every X minutes, is covered by a set of latitude–longitude–time bounding boxes of constant volume. In this case, three bounding boxes are used, and we require $\text{lat1} \times \text{lon1} \times (t2 - t1) \approx \text{lat2} \times \text{lon2} \times (t3 - t2) \approx \text{lat3} \times \text{lon3} \times (t4 - t3)$. One SQL query is then executed for each bounding box, querying the GPS events within it. These queries require no geospatial indexing in the database and are fast if the latitude–longitude–timestamp database columns are indexed.

is convenient to implement a class representing GPS trajectories, so that processing can logically be applied to instantiations of the trajectory class.

Finally, we stress that the processing of GPS data is a challenging task and represents an entire research area on its own. Due to the short development time span of the Smittestopp app, we were not able to rigorously test different processing strategies, such as map matching techniques [3, 11], filter-based approaches [9], and others (for a review, see, e.g. [15]). Rather, our goal was to develop a simple but robust solution that excludes false-positive GPS contacts within a limited development time frame.

6.3.4 Contact tracing reports

Due to the different requirements of the analysis output (see Section 6.2), the analysis pipeline can produce two report styles:

1. **Detailed style**. Information is given for each contact event between two individuals. This report is intended to be used for internal testing and debugging and contains more data than are required for pure contact tracing.
2. **Day-by-day style**. Contacts are summarized on a daily basis, showing only information that is relevant to contact tracing.

Both report styles give separate information on contacts detected by GPS and BT. By default, the report uses only contact events that match the Norwegian Institute of Public Health (NIPH) requirements, that is, with risk category 'medium', 'high', 'gps_only', or 'bt_below_15_min', as defined in Table 6.2. For debugging and internal testing, this filter can be deactivated to generate reports that show all contact

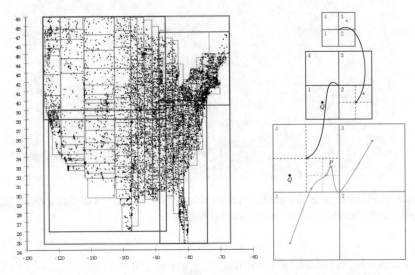

Fig. 6.5: On the left is a visualization of a geospatial database using R-trees as the tree data structure (image source: Wikipedia). The panel on the right illustrates geospatial indexing using depth 3 B-trees. Hierarchical structures allow for efficient distance queries. For example, point P, with index $(4, 2, 3)$, is not close to Q, since its index is $(4, i, \cdots)$, where, crucially, $i \neq 2$. Neither R-trees nor B-trees were used by Smittestopp, since experiments showed insufficient performance for computing trajectory intersections on large data sets. A key difference between R-/B-trees and the method described in Figure 6.4 is that the bounding boxes in R-/B-trees are computed on the database side, while the method described in Figure 6.4 computes the bounding boxes dynamically or optimally for each patient's trajectory.

events. The reports can be saved as text, in JSON format, or as HTML webpages, with static or interactive maps and plots.

GPS duration / high accuracy — BT duration	<2 min	≥ 2 min and <15 min	≥ 15 min
<30 min	not reported	bt_below_15_min	low/medium/high
≥ 30 min	gps_only	low/medium/high	low/medium/high

Table 6.2: Risk category definitions. In addition, to be included in an NIPH report, the contact event needs to contain either 1) BT contacts with a cumulative duration of over two minutes or 2) GPS contacts with an accuracy below 10 metres and a cumulative duration of at least 30 minutes.

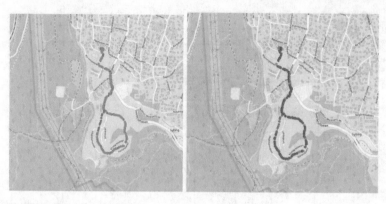

Fig. 6.6: The left panel shows the GPS trajectories of two phones during a walk. The right panel shows the identified contact points in red.

Concerning the additional risk categories *gps_only* and *bt_below_15_min* in Table 6.2, we note that, during the pre-launch testing, too few contacts were reported as *high* or *medium* risk. We suspected that one (or both) of the boundaries in the filter was too strict. Therefore two new categories (i.e. *gps_only* and *bt_below_15_min*) were introduced.

The day-by-day style report provides information on the cumulative duration, distance, and location of contacts through *points of interest*. Points of interest are determined by transport modes and amenities near the contact points and can be divided into three categories: inside (e.g. in a building or a vehicle), outside (e.g. when walking), and uncertain (when the transport modes are inconsistent). If GPS data are available for a given contact, a static map of contact trajectories is also displayed. To improve privacy, the map shows no more than necessary for contact tracing. An example of the information shown in a day-by-day style report is provided in Figure 6.7-6.12.

The detailed style reports contain information on each individual contact event. In addition to the information provided in the aggregated reports, the detailed style reports show the transport modes of the users involved in the contact and the duration of the contact spent inside and/or outside. In addition to helping determine the location, transport modes can be used to validate an actual contact by checking if two modes are consistent. The three transport modes are *still*, *on foot*, and *vehicle*. The case of a car driving past a pedestrian would not be considered a contact, because the transport modes would be *on foot* and *vehicle*. Detailed reports are only used for internal testing and validation and were not sent to NIPH.

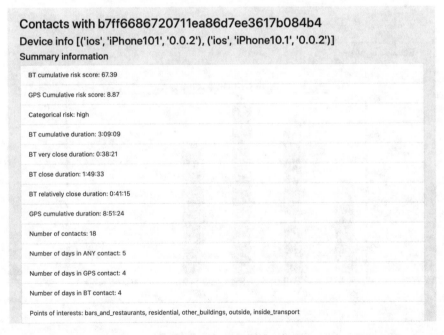

Risk report for 4577ff0a729411ea80ea42a51fad92d3
Analysis pipeline version 1.4.0
Device info [('ios', 'iPhone12.3', '0.0.4')]
Quick links:

- Contacts with b7ff6686720711ea86d7ee3617b084b4
- Contacts with 9b55b50c729411ea80ea42a51fad92d3
- Contacts with a891585872cf11ea94e20edabf845fab
- Contacts with dd84433a729411ea80ea42a51fad92d3

Fig. 6.7: Header of an example report.

Daily summary
Contact on 2020-04-06

BT cumulative duration: 0:00:00
GPS cumulative duration: 3:26:23
Number of BT contacts: 0
Number of GPS contacts: 4
Points of interests: outside, residential

Fig. 6.8: Example of a detailed daily summary.

Contacts with b7ff6686720711ea86d7ee3617b084b4
Device info [('ios', 'iPhone101', '0.0.2'), ('ios', 'iPhone10.1', '0.0.2')]
Summary information

BT cumulative risk score: 67.39
GPS Cumulative risk score: 8.87
Categorical risk: high
BT cumulative duration: 3:09:09
BT very close duration: 0:38:21
BT close duration: 1:49:33
BT relatively close duration: 0:41:15
GPS cumulative duration: 8:51:24
Number of contacts: 18
Number of days in ANY contact: 5
Number of days in GPS contact: 4
Number of days in BT contact: 4
Points of interests: bars_and_restaurants, residential, other_buildings, outside, inside_transport

Fig. 6.9: Summary information for all contacts detected with one UUID.

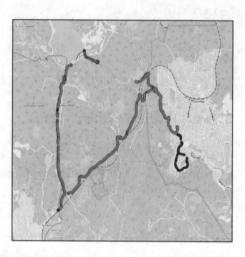

Fig. 6.10: Example of a static map generated for daily summary. The green and blue points represent user trajectories, and the red points indicate contact between users.

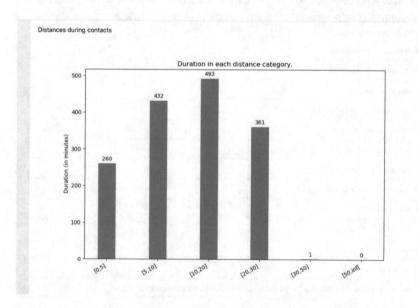

Fig. 6.11: Graph of the duration for different distances.

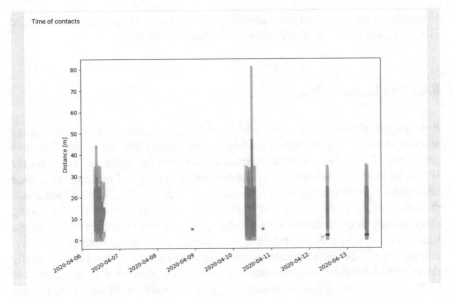

Fig. 6.12: Graph of when contact events occurred and their distances.

6.4 Smittestopp testing and validation

Since digital contact tracing is an entirely novel technology, we performed testing and validation in several phases, which allowed us to identify its strengths and weaknesses. Specifically, we performed the following three testing/validation phases:

1. **Pre-launch testing.** The goal of this study was to ensure that the solution can discover and identify close contacts, to ensure the stability and efficiency of the technology, and to adjust the parameters in the contact tracing algorithms.
2. **Real-life validation with three pilot municipalities.** The goal of the study was to acquire knowledge on how the solution can assist epidemiologists and manual contact tracers in their everyday work, to understand the challenges and benefits related to the solution from the end user perspective, and to discover technical limitations and outline directions for further improvement.
3. **Controlled testing in real-life and lab conditions.** The goal of the study was to extensively validate the technical part of the solution with respect to discoverability of true contacts (true positives) and false contacts (false positives) in real-life scenarios, as well as in lab stress testing experiments.

In addition, we closely followed other teams worldwide in terms of their validation efforts, so that we could modify our studies according to new findings.

Below we provide a detailed description of each of the studies, including the scenarios and results. It is worth mentioning that some countries working on digital tracing solutions also performed extensive testing and validation studies. Specifically, we analysed the results of the German [13] and Swiss [1] studies, which tested Google/Apple Exposure Notifications in lab and real-life scenarios.

6.4.1 Pre-launch testing

Before the launch of Smittestopp on 16 April 2020, we validated the contact tracing solution in several phases, using data from approximately 300 app testers. The main objectives of this phase were to estimate beacon proximity/distance based on the BT signal strength, evaluate phone discoverability via BT and evaluate the tracing algorithms for different types of activities (e.g. walking, driving, and indoor and outdoor activities), and understand whether GPS could be used for contact tracing alone or only in combination with BT. The results of this validation show that the tracing algorithm is quite accurate in identifying contacts if the data are available, but that the contact duration reported in the app differs from the ground truth. Usually the identified duration is slightly shorter than in reality. Additionally, the accuracy of GPS was found to be quite low in indoor locations. However, GPS seemed to provide accurate results for outdoor contacts. Moreover, this phase allowed us to understand and work on challenges related to digital tracing, as well as to specify which features could be provided to NIPH in real-life validation, as discussed above.

6.4.2 Real-life validation in testing municipalities

To validate the app as a contact tracing tool, from 27 April to 31 May, in collaboration with NIPH, we compared the results from manual and digital contact tracing in three municipalities. During the five-week test period, the uptake of the app in these municipalities was around 14%. Moreover, a rather low number of new cases, only 118, were reported during the five-week period. Of all the cases, only 31 were Smittestopp users. In total, 60 contacts were identified by Smittestopp, of which 24 (40%) were confirmed to be close contacts. Of these, 18 were also found through manual contact tracing (75%), whereas six contacts were found only through Smittestopp (25%). We also looked closely into 20 of the unconfirmed cases, identified by the app as close contacts. It appears that nine of them took place more than 48 hours before the onset of symptoms and were thus not considered true close contacts in manual tracing. The app does not consider symptom onset as one of the variables and takes into account all contacts within the past seven days, and the manual contract tracing team can then decide which contacts to notify. Another eight identified contacts had too little contact with the case (false positives). For the remaining three cases, it is difficult to verify the correctness of the digital contact tracing, since, in two cases, the phone was used by another person than the name under which it was registered and, in one case, the individual was asymptomatic.

In summary, the results of the validation demonstrate that, although Smittestopp was able to identify both contacts already identified through manual contact tracing and additional contacts not already known to the contact tracers, the risk score, adapted from the United Kingdom, required a modification to represent true contacts, since the original version was not adjusted for digital contact tracing. The results also confirm that the added value of a contact tracing app is to identify random contacts, that is, contacts not personally known to the case. Given the low numbers of cases and app users, the data collected through the municipalities was too limited to draw any further conclusions regarding the app's effectiveness in identifying contacts. Therefore, we performed additional controlled testing under real-life and lab conditions to better understand the strengths and weaknesses of digital contact tracing.

6.4.3 Controlled testing under real-life and lab conditions

In August 2020, a modified and improved version of the app was tested in two types of experiments: a stress test lab experiment and in real-life scenarios. The improvement involved enhancing the stability of the Android version of the app. The goal of the stress test was to assess the ability of the solution to discover phones in proximity when many phones are located in the same place. For more details about the test setup and phones used, see Chapter 5. The testing in real-life scenarios aimed to assess the ability of the solution to discover contacts that were either true positives or false positives in scenarios such as restaurants, shopping malls, and training centres. The detailed descriptions of the tests and their comparison with the Google/Apple solution is available in the Simula-published report on the comparison of different solutions for digital contact tracing (in Norwegian) [14]. In this section, we present only the results from real-life testing. Chapter 5 contains a detailed description of the stress test setup and results.

In the **real-life scenarios**, we tested the app's ability to discover other phones in proximity and to estimate the risk of infection if the contact was identified. In these experiments, six participants were asked to perform standard social interactions while using the testing phones in a common manner. The participants were split into three groups; in each group, one participant had an Android phone and another participant had an iOS phone. More specifically, we used the following phones: second-generation iPhone SE (two), iPhone 11, iPhone 11 Pro Max, Huawei P30 Pro, Samsung S20 5G, Sony Xperia 1, Samsung A71, and Samsung S10. The testing lasted around four hours, during which time the participants carried out different social interaction activities, such as visiting a bar, a restaurant, a training centre, or a shopping mall. Three additional phones were located in the testing areas: one with a waitress, one with a bar attendant, and one with a receptionist. The details of the protocol and scenarios are available in the report.[2]

---

[2] See https://www.simula.no/news/en-ny-runde-med-digital-smittesporing.

The participants within each group were asked to remain at one metre of each other. Each participant logged their travel details as well as information on where the phone was located. We used this information, together with the detailed protocol, to analyse the results.

Based on the protocol and the participants' logs, 66 contacts could have been identified by the technology, among which 26 should have been considered very close contacts. For our technology, we define a contact as phones being in proximity to each other (within 2 metres) for at least 10 minutes. The confusion matrix is shown in Table 6.3. Based on the results, the app has a recall of 84.6%, a precision of 73.3%, and an accuracy of 81.8%.

Real contact \ Predicted contact	Contact	No contact
Contact	84.6%	15.4%
No contact	20%	80%

Real contact \ Predicted contact	Low	High	No risk
Low	33.3%	0%	66.7%
High	10%	80%	10%
No risk	0%	0%	100%

Table 6.3: The left panel shows the confusion matrix for the discoverability of contacts: of 66 potential contacts, only 26 are close contacts and 40 are not a contact according to the NIPH definition. The right panel shows the confusion matrix for the risk identification of the contacts: of 26 real contacts, 20 are high risk and six are low risk.

In addition to discoverability, we estimated the ability of the technology to correctly assign the risk category of each contact. For simplicity and in light of the experiment design, we considered only two categories: low risk (all contacts within 2 metres for less than 25 minutes) and high risk (all contacts within 2 metres for more than 25 minutes). We again used the test protocol and the participants' logs to assign a risk category for each contact. Of 26 real contacts, 20 are expected to be high-risk contacts. The results are presented in Table 6.3.

6.5 Lessons Learned and conclusion

In this chapter, we discuss digital tracing technologies for the identification and isolation of potentially close contacts of an infected individual. We show that the technology is feasible, but the main prerequisite for its validation and success is reasonable uptake in a population and close collaboration with epidemiologists. Issues related to defining an epidemiologically meaningful ranking of contacts remain open. We believe that a large validation trial with real-life scenarios is necessary to find the optimal risk score function. A big challenge in the validation of the digital tracing technology is that access to the collected data is very limited. In the case of Smittestopp, the technology was developed using a test data set but applied to real data, which are of completely different size, with much greater variation, leading to challenges related to computational efficiency. How to validate a digital tracing tool efficiently while complying with privacy and security regulations is not yet fully understood.

Our work shows that both GPS and BT data are important for obtaining a better understanding of how digital contact tracing works and illustrates their usefulness to epidemiologists. BT data allow proximity events to be identified, whereas GPS data provides contextualization for the contacts found. We believe that once the digital tracing technology is validated, GPS data can be excluded and the technology can be based only on BT data.

References

[1] SwissCovid exposure score calculation, 11 September 2020.

[2] R. Bayer and E. McCreight. Organization and maintenance of large ordered indices. In *Proceedings of the 1970 ACM SIGFIDET (Now SIGMOD) Workshop on Data Description, Access and Control*, SIGFIDET '70, page 107–141, New York, NY, USA, 1970. Association for Computing Machinery.

[3] M. Bierlaire, J. Chen, and J. Newman. A probabilistic map matching method for smartphone GPS data. *Transportation Research Part C: Emerging Technologies*, 26:78–98, 2013.

[4] L. Bourouiba, E. Dehandschoewercker, and J. W. Bush. Violent expiratory events: on coughing and sneezing. *Journal of Fluid Mechanics*, 745:537–563, 2014.

[5] G. M. Djuknic and R. E. Richton. Geolocation and assisted GPS. *Computer*, 34(2):123–125, 2001.

[6] L. Ferretti, C. Wymant, M. Kendall, L. Zhao, A. Nurtay, L. Abeler-Dörner, M. Parker, D. Bonsall, and C. Fraser. Quantifying SARS-CoV-2 transmission suggests epidemic control with digital contact tracing. *Science*, 368(6491), 2020.

[7] A. Guttman. R-trees: A dynamic index structure for spatial searching. In *Proceedings of the 1984 ACM SIGMOD International Conference on Management of Data*, SIGMOD '84, page 47–57, New York, NY, USA, 1984. Association for Computing Machinery.

[8] R. Hinch, W. Probert, A. Nurtay, M. Kendall, C. Wymant, M. Hall, and C. Fraser. Effective configurations of a digital contact tracing app: A report to nhsx. en. In:(Apr. 2020). Available here. url: https://github. com/BDI-pathogens/covid-19_instant_tracing/blob/master/Report, 2020.

[9] W.-C. Lee and J. Krumm. Trajectory preprocessing. In *Computing with spatial trajectories*, pages 3–33. Springer, 2011.

[10] D. J. Leith and S. Farrell. Coronavirus contact tracing: Evaluating the potential of using bluetooth received signal strength for proximity detection. 2020.

[11] Y. Lou, C. Zhang, Y. Zheng, X. Xie, W. Wang, and Y. Huang. Map-matching for low-sampling-rate GPS trajectories. In *Proceedings of the 17th ACM SIGSPA-TIAL international conference on advances in geographic information systems*, pages 352–361, 2009.

[12] K. Merry and P. Bettinger. Smartphone GPS accuracy study in an urban environment. *PloS one*, 14(7):e0219890, 2019.

[13] S. Meyer, T. Windisch, N. Witt, and D. Dziebela. Google exposure notification API testing (Germany). URL: https://github.com/corona-warn-app/cwa-documentation/blob/master/2020_06_24_Corona_API_measurements.pdf, June 2020.

[14] Simula Research Laboratory and Simula Metropolitan. Sammenligning av alternative løsninger for digital smittesporing, 2020.

[15] R. Wu, G. Luo, J. Shao, L. Tian, and C. Peng. Location prediction on trajectory data: A review. *Big data mining and analytics*, 1(2):108–127, 2018.

Chapter 7
Data aggregation and anonymization for mathematical modeling and epidemiological studies

Are Magnus Bruaset, Glenn Terje Lines and Joakim Sundnes

Abstract An important secondary purpose of the Smittestopp development was to provide aggregated data sets describing mobility and social interactions in Norway's population. The data were to be used to monitor the effect of government regulations and recommendations, provide input to advanced computational models to predict the pandemic's spread, and provide input to fundamental epidemiology research. In this chapter we describe the challenges and technical solutions of Smittestopp's data aggregation, as well as preliminary results from the time period when the app was active. We first give a detailed overview of the requirements, specifying the types of data to be collected and the level of spatial and temporal aggregation. We then proceed to describe the concepts for anonymization via k-anonymity and ε-differential privacy (ε-DP), and the technical solutions for collecting and aggregating data from the database. In particular, we present details of how GPS- and Bluetooth events were mapped to geographical regions and points of interest, and the solutions employed for efficient data retrieval and processing. The preliminary results demonstrate how the recorded GPS- and Bluetooth events match with expected temporal and spatial variations in mobility and social interactions, and indicate the usefulness of the aggregated data as a tool for pandemic monitoring and research. One of the main criticisms of Smittestopp concerns the centralized storage of individuals' movements, even if such data were used and presented only at an aggregated and anonymized level. In this chapter, we also outline a completely different approach, where the GPS data do not leave the user's phone but are, instead, pre-processed to a much

A. M. Bruaset
Department of High performance Computing , Simula Research Laboratory,
e-mail: arem@simula.no

G. T. Lines
Department of Computational Physiology, Simula Research Laboratory
e-mail: glennli@simula.no

J. Sundnes
Department of Computational Physiology, Simula Research Laboratory
e-mail: sundnes@simula.no

© The Author(s) 2022
A. Elmokashfi et al. (eds.), *Smittestopp – A Case Study on Digital Contact Tracing*,
Simula SpringerBriefs on Computing 11, https://doi.org/10.1007/978-3-031-05466-2_7

higher level of privacy before being dispatched to a server-side data aggregation algorithm. This approach, which would make the app significantly less intrusive, is made possible by recent advances in determining close contacts from Bluetooth data, either by a revised Smittestopp algorithm or by means of the Google/Apple Exposure Notification framework.

7.1 Introduction

The aim of this chapter is to explain the reasoning and the strategies behind the aggregation of Smittestopp's data in space and time, to provide high-level information about population dynamics and the spread of disease. For instance, this information could shed light on understanding how, when and where close contacts occur, and could be used to understand how imposed interventions, such as advice on social distancing and changes to public transportation patterns, are met by the public. The techniques described were under implementation and subject to preliminary tests when Smittestopp's development was put on hold. The implementation was therefore not completed or fully deployed in Smittestopp's production system. Based on the gathered experiences regarding scalability, we also present ideas for a distributed aggregation scheme. If implemented, this scheme would also provide improved protection of app users' privacy.

7.2 Data requirements and privacy

As described earlier, the aggregated data sets from Smittestopp were meant to serve several purposes. First, the aggregated data from the app would provide continuous information on movements and interactions in the population during the pandemic, and would be used to monitor how various restrictions and government interventions impact social interactions and, in turn, the spread of the disease. Second, it would provide potentially valuable input to the predictive epidemiology models that inform political decisions and healthcare planning [7]. Data from the app would provide such information on a daily basis, unlike the three- to four-week delay between a change in social interactions and a visible change in COVID-19 hospital cases. This unique and detailed data would also be a resource for long-term epidemiology research, to improve prediction and insight in preparation for future pandemics. Finally, the aggregated data would be used to provide statistics and information to the public, to increase knowledge and awareness in the general population. To serve these different purposes, a requirement list was prepared by the Norwegian Institute of Public Health (NIPH), which specified the following four aggregated data sets with varying levels of detail.

Data set 1: Individual-based data on the movement patterns and behaviour of app users. The first data set was to be collected for anonymized individuals, with tables summarizing key numbers for each individual app user. The temporal resolution would be one day, while the spatial aggregation would be at the municipality level. The municipality of Oslo is treated as a special case, with aggregation for each district (*bydel*). A more detailed description of the geographical units used for aggregation is provided in Section 7.3, below. For each municipality and each day, a table is produced, with one row for each app user, and the following columns: travel on foot (total in minutes); travel by vehicle (total in minutes); minutes spent indoors, outdoors, and in particular locations, including grocery shops, kindergartens, schools, offices, hospitals, parks, and residences; and, finally, the total travel distance.

All individual data items would be extracted from the GPS data of the individual app users. Anonymity and privacy would be preserved by anonymizing all app users and ensuring that every table contains at least k rows, as described in more detail below. For units with fewer than k app users, the aggregation would be moved to the next level of spatial resolution, that is, from the municipality to the county level. With a typical k value of 20, it is unlikely that this additional aggregation is needed, since all municipalities are expected to have far more than 20 app users.

Data set 2: Location-based data set highlighting the exposure of individual locations to the population. The main purpose of the second data set is to inform about potential disease transmission and guide government regulations and recommendations. Locations of interest are extracted from OpenStreetMap (OSM), and include hospitals, schools, shops, and bus/train stops, etc., and are stored in local files containing a unique ID, name, municipality, type of location, position, and geometry. The geographical data and algorithms to collect them are described in more detail below. The resulting local database of points of interest (POIs) is combined with the GPS data from Smittestopp to count the number of visitors to each location and the time they spend there. As for the first data set, privacy is guarded by lumping any location with fewer than k visits together with nearby locations of the same type. The anonymity-preserving aggregation step is likely to be more relevant for this data set, than for Data set 1, since many locations can have fewer than 20 visitors per day.

Data set 3: Bluetooth contacts quantifying the level of interaction in the population. The Bluetooth contact data from Smittestopp is a unique data set for quantifying contacts that could potentially transmit disease. Based on Bluetooth pairings between phones with the Smittestopp app, we count all critical contacts, that is, contacts with an estimated duration of more than 15 minutes and a distance of less than 2 metres. The number of contacts is aggregated at the municipality and district levels, with a temporal resolution of one to several hours. To normalize the data to the number of app users, we also count the number of app users belonging to each geographical unit on a given day:

$$PM_1, PM_2, \ldots PM_{355+15},$$

where PM_i is the number of app users on a given day in municipality i, for $i \leq 355$, or in the corresponding district in Oslo when $i = 356, \ldots, 370$. Similar numbers $PC_1, PC_2, \ldots PC_{11}$ are recorded at the county level.

Data set 4: summary statistics on the number of contacts and movement patterns. The final data set is intended to provide summary statistics on contacts and movement patterns to the public. The data are aggregated from the three other data sets into statistical indicators suitable for public use.

7.2.1 Privacy-preserving techniques

Recorded details on where individuals move around and who they meet can potentially be misused in the hands of a malicious third party and therefore constitute a significant privacy risk. This aspect of Smittestopp was a major concern for all parties involved: the politicians mandating the Smittestopp's development, NIPH as the system owner, and Simula as the developer of the technology. However, in the face of the thousands of casualties in Southern Europe, the national explosion of COVID-19 cases when Norwegian tourists returned from winter break in the Alps, and the potential of acutely overloading health services and running short on medical supplies, the government found the threat of COVID-19 to outweigh the time-limited privacy risk through Smittestopp's implementation. The government therefore provided the necessary legal basis [6]. The gravity of the situation and the implicit urgency to design and implement a digital tool capable of fighting the disease's spread were strongly felt by all the participants in the development process.

One fundamental principle dictating the aggregation of Smittestopp data was that no researchers or analysts are allowed direct access to the raw data. All aggregation had to be carried out once and for all on the incoming data, typically in batches once or twice per day, through totally automated scripts that are run inside a secure environment in the Azure cloud. Only aggregated and anonymized information would be made accessible for a group of authorized personnel and researchers. Moreover, the raw data going into the aggregation pipeline had no user-specific information attached other than a randomly assigned tag that would be unique for a user for a short period, in order to combine data items correctly in the aggregation algorithms. Such tags were removed in the data aggregation procedures. The details of this architecture are discussed in Chapter 3.

Data thresholds and k-anonymity. An immediate and simple approach to reducing the privacy risk was to use sufficiently coarse spatial and temporal levels, such that a large group of people map their individual actions to the same aggregated event. For instance, although only one or two people might be waiting for a bus at the Sanatoriet bus stop at 10:29 on a given day, there might be several tens of people waiting for a bus somewhere in the Nordre Aker city quarter between 10:00 and 12:00 that day. Therefore, the coarseness of the latter event shields people's privacy more than the first detailed event mentioned. As explained in Section 7.2, one would record such aggregated events *only* if sufficiently many people (k) take part, say, $k > 20$. Otherwise, the event would be blanked from the overall statistics by being labeled "-". The use of this type of threshold is common in statistical reviews, such as the reports provided by Statistics Norway or similar national agencies in other countries, or when reporting on medical trials. It is also essential to treat data outliers, either by deleting entries with outlier values or clamping these values to the closest "safe" values.

The threshold-based approach mentioned above, which was under implementation for Smittestopp, is related to the concept of k-anonymity. Assume you have a data set where each entry lists the values of some features of an individual, say, age and nationality. If each entry in this data set is identical to $k - 1$ other entries in the same data set, the data set is said to have the property of k-anonymity [8]. Clearly, any personal identifiers such as names and ID numbers must be blanked from the data set. Then numeric values, such as age, must be bracketed in intervals that are sufficiently large to have at least k entries each. At the same time, non-numeric features must also have at least k identical entries. This can be achieved by aggregating the values into a combined value, for instance, mapping all entries with a nationality belonging to a Nordic country to the wider characteristic of 'Nordic'. Finally, the combinations of all the values of the represented features – age and nationality in this case – must have at least k entries. For instance, it is not sufficient to have at least k entries marked as Norwegian and at least k entries belonging to the age group 20–29 years if there is only a single Norwegian in that age group. By construction, this approach is most relevant for low-dimensional data sets. Moreover, it might be necessary to delete entries or add fictitious entries in order to maintain k-anonymity and simultaneously avoid aggregation to so coarse levels of feature values that they do not carry any useful information. Generally, the generation of a k-anonymous version of a data set is an NP-complete problem, but there exist implementations of several approximate algorithms designed for practical use.

Rigorous anonymization in a mathematical sense is impossible to achieve; that is, it is impossible to guarantee that an individual cannot be identified from a data set when this set can be combined with any other, known or unknown, data source at some past, current, or future time. This has been demonstrated in several studies. For instance, it is well know that k-anonymity can be compromised by data homogeneity [2], or when there is additional information from other sources [5]. However, it is always a question of whether the deduced information truly threatens anonymity; to be such a threat, the data must reveal information that is not previously generally known from any existing and available data source.

Improved protection through ε-differential privacy. Despite the lack of rigorous anonymity, it is possible to achieve reasonable levels of anonymization by careful design, thus reducing the privacy risks to acceptable levels. When planning the data aggregation strategies of Smittestopp, we consulted the relevant literature, as well as experts in Norway and abroad. We also closely examined the feedback from the panel of experts assigned with the task of evaluating Smittestopp' technology [4]. Based on this combined input, we concluded that the two most relevant approaches to anonymization would be k-anonymity, as outlined above, and ε-DP . While k-anonymity was under implementation when Smittestopp's development was halted, the implementation of ε-DP was at the planning stage.

The essence of ε-DP is to give each individual represented in a data set as much privacy as if that individual's data were removed from the set. This is achieved by injecting random noise into the data set. To illustrate the concept, consider a survey where each individual is asked to respond yes or no to a sensitive question. Once the true answer is given, an algorithm draws a random number between zero and one. If this number is less than 0.5, the true answer is passed to the data set. If the value is at or above 0.5, a second random number is drawn. If this second number is less than 0.5, the value yes is inserted into the data set, and otherwise the value no is injected. For real applications, more sophisticated implementations would be used, and the parameters of the algorithm would be tuned to yield a prescribed level of privacy as indicated by the value of ε [1]. This method has been developed through both academic and industrial research. For instance, it has received substantial support from Microsoft,[1] and Apple is one of the technology companies that have been embracing ε-DP as a means to protect their users' privacy.[2] While promising, it is also well known that ε-DP is no magic recipe that always guarantees full privacy [9]. In particular, its performance in terms of privacy protection depends strongly on the choice of ε, and some implementations in use have been criticized for using overly large values. Still, ε-DP remains one of the, if not *the*, best approach currently available.

Implementation of ε-DP in Smittestopp. Up until the decision of halting Smittestopp's development, considerable effort was made in optimizing the script-based data extraction and processing, including the proper use of data thresholds (see Section 7.5). These computationally demanding procedures had to be in place before we could add the most sophisticated privacy protection in terms of ε-DP . Therefore, no data are available on the performance of ε-DP in the Smittestopp case, or on exactly how the data manipulation implied by ε-DP would affect the quality of the aggregated data. Similarly, the project halted before it was possible to determine an appropriate value for ε. As many other parts of Smittestopp's development, the work on ε-DP would have been at the frontiers of research. Since the development was halted, this research has not yet been further pursued.

---

[1] See *New differential privacy platform co-developed with Harvard's OpenDP unlocks data while safeguarding privacy*, 24 June 2020, at https://blogs.microsoft.com/on-the-issues/2020/06/24/differential-privacy-harvard-opendp/.

[2] See *Learning with Privacy at Scale*, December 2017, at https://docs-assets.developer.apple.com/ml-research/papers/learning-with-privacy-at-scale.pdf.

7.3 Geographical units and points of interest

All the specified data sets rely on various forms of geographical and geometrical data. All spatial data aggregation would be performed relative to standard geographical units, such as districts, municipalities, and counties, and the mapping of GPS events to these units relies on their geometrical data. Similarly, the POI analysis naturally relies on geometrical information about the POIs to map app user trajectories to the various locations. For reasons of efficiency, the geographical data needed to be fetched, pre-processed, and stored locally for use in the data analysis.

Norway is divided into 11 counties, which are again subdivided into municipalities, of which there are 356 in total. Each municipality is further divided into parts (*delområder*, 1,558 in total) and, finally, basic statistical units (BSUs, or *grunnkretser*, 14,097 in mainland Norway) at the finest level. Each geographical unit has a unique numerical identifier, which is two digits long for the counties, with two extra digits added for each subsequent layer. For example, the Torgalmenningen BSU has the eight-digit ID 46010129. It belongs to the *delområde* Bergen Sentrum, with ID 460101, the municipality of Bergen (ID 4601) and the county of Vestland (ID 46). Oslo is treated as a special case, since it is both a county and a municipality. Here, the municipality level is used instead to represent city districts (*bydeler*).

Geographical information for all these units was downloaded from the publicly available repository geonorge.no as Geography Markup Language (GML) files. The geometric representation used in the original format is very general and verbose and, for efficiency, needed to be simplified, such that each unit could be represented as a single polygon. The final result was stored locally in a JSON file for later use in the data aggregation and analysis.

Data sets 1 and 2 specified above both rely on geographical information about POIs. For Data set 1, we want to count the time spent by individuals in locations such as grocery stores, schools, and parks, while Data set 2 provides a list of the same location types and specifies their total exposure to the population. The Overpass API to OSM provides an excellent resource for extracting such information and acts as a database that supports queries based on polygons and bounding box data. Data are returned in a dictionary-like format, providing for each POI a unique identifier, a name, a type, and various relevant tags. Depending on the type of POI, geometrical information is provided in the form of its centre coordinates, bounding box, or the polygonal data for its boundary. With such information available, GPS trajectories from Smittestopp can be used to estimate the number of visits and time spent at the various POIs.

There are two main ways to access and use OSM data. The first is to use the data as an online database, which is queried whenever we need information about a POI, thereby ensuring that the most recent information is used for all POIs. However, such queries to the database are fairly slow, particularly queries using polygonal data, and since the data sets include tens of thousands of POIs and are based on the GPS trajectories of hundreds of thousands of users, basing the entire analysis on database queries is not feasible. Furthermore, the frequency of updates in OSM is relatively slow and, on a time scale of weeks to a few months, the information is approximately static. These considerations motivated the second approach, which is based on batch processing OSM queries and storing the POI information locally in a simplified format. These local files contain only essential information, that is, the POI name, type, and geometrical information, and are used for processing the GPS data from the app.

For the first version of the aggregation pipeline, one file was created for each POI type, containing the name of the POI and the geometry specified by the bounding box. The use of polygonal data would obviously allow for more accurate results, and detailed polygonal geometries are available for most POIs. However, as discussed above, computational efficiency was a high priority throughout the development of the data aggregation pipeline, because of the huge volumes of data involved and strict 24-hour processing time limit.

7.4 Data analysis and preliminary results

As described in Section 7.1, the Smittestopp app was put on hold and the collected data deleted before the data aggregation was put into full use. Therefore, no aggregated data sets were ever produced from the full-scale *production* database. However, most of the algorithms for aggregation and analysis were implemented and tested on a smaller development database, and limited trial runs were performed on the full database in the final days before the data were deleted. In this section, we describe some of the algorithms used and their Python implementation, as well as some preliminary results from the initial trial runs.

Data were retrieved by accessing the SQL server via a small set of access functions. The code below is a simple example of usage, where the function `getGPSWithinGrunnkrets` is used to extract all GPS events recorded by the app in a single day within a single BSU:

```
from corona.data import connect_to_azure_database
import pandas as pd

db = connect_to_azure_database()
key = "03012305"
date_from = "2020-04-27"
date_to = "2020-04-28"
query = f"select * from getGPSWithinGrunnkrets('{key}' ,\
'{date_from}', '{date_to}')"
df = pd.read_sql(query, con=db)
db.close()
```

Connection to the database is first established through the connect call. For efficiency reasons and unlike in this example, the connection would typically be kept open for multiple calls, and a new connection only created if the previous one was broken. Data were returned as pandas frames, with one line per event. Field types varied with the type of query issued.

Computational efficiency was an important consideration throughout the aggregation pipeline's development, and a recurring question concerned the amount of analysis that should be performed on the server side versus the client side. One

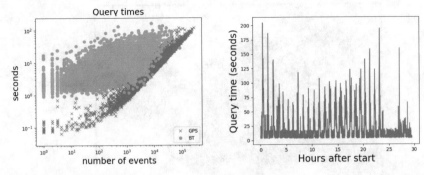

Fig. 7.1: The left panel shows the time spent on data retrieval for the two data types BT and GPS. Data are from one full day and from all the BSUs of Norway. Each data point represents one BSU. The *x*-axis shows the number of matching rows in the database. The right panel shows the query times as a function of runtime (summed over both types). Hourly congestion is evident, as well as a 24-hour cycle.

strategy is to limit the need to move data off the server, by carrying out as much aggregation as possible inside the SQL access functions. The other extreme would be to extract all necessary data from the server using the simplest possible queries and to carry out all aggregation and post-processing in Python on the client side. Although the issue was not fully explored, our preliminary trial indicated that the optimal solution is a balanced approach between minimizing data movement and avoiding excessive computations on the server side. In Figure 7.1, we show the time spent retrieving data from the server. These are data from a single day and from all 14,097 BSUs. With the current implementation, the majority of time is spent on data retrieval. Data size is only loosely correlated with waiting times, and some of this can be explained by congestion on the server. The panel on the right shows the variation in query times as a function of time. The processing times for the data generated in a 24-hour window would easily exceed 24 hours, which is, of course, not acceptable performance. The main reason was that the database server was unable to keep up with the combined load of influx of new data and the high numbers of queries generated by both the contact tracing and the data aggregation pipelines. This problem could be alleviated by a more distributed approach, as discussed towards the end of this chapter.

7.4.1 Mapping GPS events to BSUs and POIs

Data were to be aggregated from the smallest geographical unit, the BSU. A natural way to perform the analysis was to loop over all 14,097 BSUs in Norway and collect the relevant GPS and Bluetooth events based on the location coordinates. The first method we evaluated was the query function `getWithinPolygon`. This

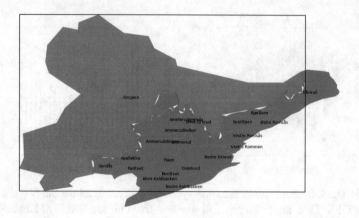

Fig. 7.2: Example of a bounding box as a proxy for a polygon (the red area) failing badly. Most of the neighbouring district (the green area) is also included.

method only worked for certain polygons, and it turned out that the query length was limited to 4, 000 characters. Polygons with many points would exceed this limit and cause the call to fail silently, returning zero events. The problem was circumvented by downsampling all polygons to fewer than 150 points, which was sufficient to stay within the maximum query length. The downsampling was performed using `Polygon.simplify` from the Shapely library, which performed the downsampling very well, and no significant accuracy was lost due to this simplification.

In the end, however, it turned out that `getWithinPolygon` was too slow for the aggregation pipeline, even with the modified polygons. Instead, a simplified query function was implemented, `getWithinBB`, that avoided the inside polygon test and instead returned data points with coordinates inside a given bounding box. This alone could not replace the more accurate polygon test, since large areas would be erroneously included in each BSU, sometimes adding a huge amount of extra data (see Figure 7.2 for an example).

When we used `getWithinBB`, the filtering was instead performed in the Python script on the client side, again relying on the Shapely library. Specifically, we employed the `contains` function in the module `shapely.vectorized`, which could work on a complete data set at once, and we thus avoided explicit loops on the Python side. An example of usage is shown below.

```
def polygon_vectorized_filter_df(df, coords):
    """ Returns subset of df that actually
        belongs to the given polygon. """
    polygon = shapely.Polygon(coords)
    x, y = df.loc[:,'longitude'], df.loc[:,'latitude']
    mask = shapely.vectorized.contains(polygon, x, y)
    return df.loc[mask,:].copy()
```

This function call had a negligible computational cost, and the mapping of events to the correct BSUs no longer represented a bottleneck. However, the solution was by no means optimal, since large amounts of data would be moved from the server only to be thrown away by the filtering on the client side. A further improvement was implemented in which the data points were tagged with the correct BSUs already upon insertion, thus avoiding the polygon test altogether at the time of query. An example call is included in the first code segment in Section 7.4.

The core of the POI processing is similar to the mapping to BSUs and involves computing intersections between app users' GPS trajectories and the various POIs. These computations would be performed as a post-processing step applied to the aggregated data at the BSU or municipality level. To account for the variable GPS accuracy, we viewed each point in a user's trajectory as a square bounding box, with the measured coordinates in its centre and sides equal to two times the given GPS accuracy. For reasons of efficiency, the initial version of the pipeline also represented the POI geometries by their bounding boxes. The mapping of GPS coordinates to POIs was then reduced to computing intersections between bounding boxes, which involves only a comparison of (at most) four numbers and a few logical operations. Using the full polygonal data from OSM for the POIs would obviously produce more accurate results, but this could become a potential bottleneck when mapping tens of thousands of POIs to the trajectories of millions of app users. The following example function takes as input a data frame with the app user's trajectories, a dictionary of POIs, and the GPS accuracy in metres, and it performs a partially vectorized computation of all the bounding box interactions.

```python
def get_intersections_vectorized(df, poi_bbs, distanceInMeters):
    contacts = []
    if len(df)==0:
        return contacts

    lat = df.latitude.values; lon = df.longitude.values

    latRadian = lat*np.pi/180
    degLatKm = 110.574235
    degLongKm = 110.572833 * np.cos(latRadian)
    deltaLat = distanceInMeters / 1000.0 / degLatKm
    deltaLong = distanceInMeters / 1000.0 / degLongKm
    lon_min = lon - deltaLong; lon_max = lon + deltaLong
    lat_min = lat - deltaLat; lat_max = lat + deltaLat

    for poi in poi_bbs:
        poi_lon_min = poi_bbs[poi]['minlon']
        poi_lon_max = poi_bbs[poi]['maxlon']
        lon_sep = np.logical_or(lon_min>poi_lon_max, lon_max<poi_lon_min)

        poi_lat_min = poi_bbs[poi]['minlat']
        poi_lat_max = poi_bbs[poi]['maxlat']
        lat_sep = np.logical_or(lat_min>poi_lat_max, lat_max<poi_lat_min)

        intersection = np.logical_not(np.logical_or(lat_sep, lon_sep))
        index = np.nonzero(intersection)[0]
        contacts.append(len(index))

    return contacts
```

This code obviously holds potential for further optimization, but it is already considerably more efficient than the most basic version based on two nested loops and polygonal data for the POIs. The non-vectorized loop over the POI dictionary might be the most natural candidate for further refinement, but the typical POI dictionary has only a few thousand entries, which is three to four orders of magnitude smaller

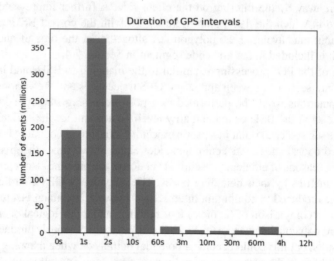

Fig. 7.3: Nearby GPS events are merged into a single event. The figure shows the resulting distribution of event durations.

than the data frame of users' GPS coordinates. Vectorizing the loop over coordinate points is therefore clearly the most important improvement.

Estimating users' dwelling location. To quantify movement patterns, we wanted to know the BSU in which each app user lived. The basic idea was to use app users' nighttime locations according to the GPS position as a proxy for this. A complicating factor was that there was often no signal in the middle of the night, either because of signal merging (see Figure 7.3) or because, more critically, users' phones were switched off. To address this issue, we used a criterion where the user had to be present in the BSU both during the late evening and early morning. More specifically, there had to be at least one GPS event between 21:00 and 2:00 and at least one event between 4:00 and 8:00. The implementation details are shown in the code segment below. This criterion generated a good correlation between the estimated number of app users in a given BSU and the official population count according to Statistics Norway. Figure 7.4 shows a scatter plot for this. For BSUs with very small populations, overestimates can be caused by people staying overnight at a location other than their official home address, for instance, due to changes in everyday life caused by restricted access to offices and universities during the pandemic.

Since Python is an interpreted language, it was important to utilize precompiled functions from the libraries as much as possible, to avoid computational bottlenecks. Avoiding loops in Python through vectorized calls is an important technique in this respect. The approach is illustrated by the code segment below, which implements the algorithm outlined above for estimating the number of app users in a given BSU.

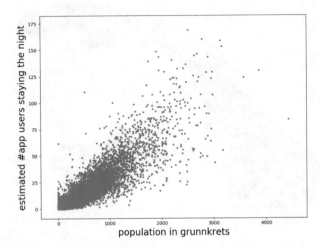

Fig. 7.4: This figure shows the population of the BSUs (or *grunnkretser*) on the horizontal axis and the estimated number of app users on the vertical axis. The correlation between between the two is 0.917.

```
# df is a Pandas data frame with one line for each GPS event
T = pd.DatetimeIndex(df['timefrom'])
# H will be a numpy array containing hour-part of timestamp
H = T.hour

# Estimate number of dwellers for this dataframe.
# True for all events after 21.00 or before 02.00:
start_blip = np.nonzero((H>21)+(H<2))
# True for all events between 04.00 and 08.00:
end_blip = np.nonzero((H>4)*(H<8))
# Find all users seen in the evening:
uuid_start = set(df.iloc[start_blip]['uuid'])
# Find all users seen in the morning:
uuid_end =   set(df.iloc[end_blip]['uuid'])
# Take the intersections to find those staying the night:
dwellers = uuid_start.intersection(uuid_end)
num_dwellers = len(dwellers)
```

An interesting use of the dwelling location estimates is to quantify regional differences in app uptake, computed as the ratios between the estimated numbers of users and the population count for each municipality. A map is shown in Figure 7.5, where dark red corresponds to an uptake of 20%. The real uptake numbers are higher, since only about 50% of the app users were captured using the criterion above. In addition, the calculation was based on a single day of data, whereas counting GPS events from several days would probably have captured more users. It is still interesting to note that some of the outliers (e.g. Hol) had local outbreaks at the time of the app's introduction and were presumably populations with an increased incentive to install the app.

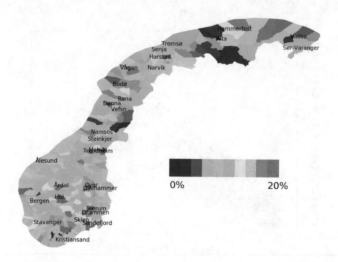

Fig. 7.5: The map shows the app uptake in Norwegian municipalities, that is, the numbers of app users relative to their population. The number of users is estimated based on their nighttime location.

Movement and contact pattern using GPS and Bluetooth data. To quantify movement during the daytime, GPS data for each BSU were aggregated into histograms with a one hour resolution. To correct for differences in population and the fact there are generally more events during daytime, each BSU was normalized to the total number of events over the entire 24 hour period. This normalization allowed us to identify areas that were relatively more active during certain parts of the day. Figure 7.6 shows the activity level in Oslo between 10:00 and 14:00, showing clearly increased daytime activity in the central regions compared to the suburbs. While this result is not very surprising, it clearly shows how GPS-based mobility mapping can be a valuable tool for health authorities and politicians, for instance, to evaluate the effects of movement restrictions and recommendations on social distancing.

The potential utility of the Bluetooth contact data was demonstrated by an interesting event on Friday, 5 June 2020. On this date, a large group of people gathered in front of the National Parliament in Oslo. With media images showing a large crowd of people standing close together, it was obvious that the event would create a local increase in the number of close contacts. Figure 7.7 shows the number of registered Bluetooth contacts in the relevant BSU, compared with the same data from one week earlier. The obvious spike in the curve coincides with the time of the event and demonstrates the ability of the Bluetooth contact data to capture events of increased interaction.

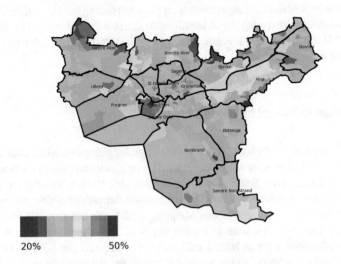

20%   50%

Fig. 7.6: Ratio of GPS events between 10:00 and 14:00 in relation to the entire day. Red signifies high daytime activity.

7.5 Distributed data aggregation

As mentioned in Section 7.3, one particular challenge in the data aggregation is in processing all incoming GPS events fast enough to keep up with the volume of con-

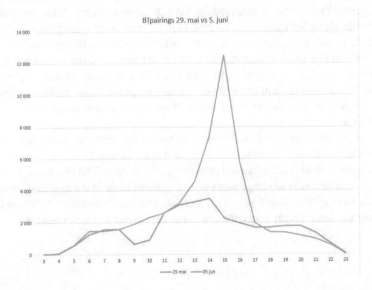

Fig. 7.7: Number of Bluetooth contacts registered in front of the National Parliament. The grey curve is from the day of a major demonstration, while the orange curve is for the same weekday (Friday) one week earlier.

tinuously acquired data. This processing applies to placing events in their respective BSUs, potentially mapping these locations to coarser spatial units, identifying the type of POI for each relevant event, and aggregating the time of each event to a time interval of reasonable coarseness.

7.5.1 Computational challenges

The BSUs are defined by more than $14,000$ irregular polygons, while coarser spatial units are either a cluster of neighbouring BSUs or a more complex construction that involves dividing some BSUs, for instance, to match the border of a municipality. In addition, there are several tens of thousands smaller polygons describing relevant POIs such as schools, kindergartens, shopping malls, and bus stops. While POIs are indexed by BSU identificators to reduce the workload, there is a need to perform all these calculations for at least 1 million events received per hour. It should also be added that these calculations would cater only for the simplest types of analysis defined by the requirements presented in Section 7.2. These analyses would answer simple questions regarding population dynamics, such as observing how current pandemic interventions affect the density of people at bus stops, shopping malls, and so forth, during the day. More advanced statistical measures, for instance, combining location data with information about close contacts extracted from Bluetooth data to better describe how people interact in the population, would further increase the computational burden.

When carrying out this processing server-side, the processing time of the last period (e.g. 24 hours) of harvested data must be *significantly* less than the length of the period in order to be prepared for the next period's batch. This time buffer is essential to allow for unforeseen delays, such as temporary disruptions to the data ingestion, insufficient allocation of computational resources in the cloud, or failed computations that need to be rerun. Due to the sensitivity of the raw data gathered, which calls for data aggregation to take place in a securely closed environment without human interaction, there are essentially no possibilities for conducting off-line processing or for using any trial and error approach. It must simply work, reliably and on time.

The experience gathered in Smittestopp's data aggregation shows that, for the server-side processing to work, as large a portion of the processing as possible must be batch-oriented and implemented in the actual SQL calls. The overhead of the data selection and access is too large to allow fine-grained logic in the aggregation scripts to repeatedly call SQL functions on smaller data chunks. Moreover, the Python-based scripting must use vector operations as much as possible to work efficiently.

7.5.2 Improving scalability through massive parallelism

Even with clever use of Python and SQL, the computational challenge posed by the data aggregation is large. It would scale badly when more app users are added, unless the frequency of the data acquisition and therefore the precision of the measurements are significantly reduced. From this perspective, it is natural to consider a divide and conquer strategy by devising a method that works in a widely distributed way. Observing that modern smartphones are essentially handheld computers with significant computational power, it would be tempting to pool together hundreds of thousands, or even millions, of these devices' computational resources to become a virtual supercomputer. In the language of high-performance computing, this would be an example of extremely massive parallelism, although with much less communication capacity than for a real supercomputer. However, as long as each phone computes only on data collected by that particular phone, and this computation involves communication only between that phone and the cloud-based server, we have a setup with trivial parallelism and very simple communication patterns.

Geographical units. This distributed computation could work as follows. The Smittestopp app stores timestamped GPS coordinates frequently, as before. Using a simple lattice grid of longitude and latitude values covering the whole country, combined with precomputed bounding boxes for each BSU stored on the phone, it is easy to compile a list of the relevant geographical units where the particular phone might have been over a specific period. Let us assume that this process is carried out once a day, at midnight, processing all GPS events recorded for the last 24 hours. The phone then asks the server to provide the polygons for only the relevant BSUs, and the phone can match the recorded GPS events to these polygons to accurately identify the BSUs where the phone was during the previous period. Most people will not move around that much on a daily basis, meaning that the data access can be further optimized by caching the BSUs in use over a few days. Overall, this approach is similar to level of detail algorithms for data visualization or the way Google Maps downloads only the map data close to your actual location to save communication bandwidth. The key is to minimize the amount of data that needs to be compared to GPS events and the amount of communication needed to obtain the data.

Adding POIs Obviously, this approach can be used for any other definition of geographical regions as well, so long as these regions are described by one or more polygons, with GPS coordinates for their corners. In particular, this approach can treat clusters of BSUs as a region, or counties and municipalities. Once the phone has identified the actual BSUs affected, it can ask the server to provide the polygons for all relevant POIs within these BSUs. The same type of calculation can then be carried out based on these polygons and the recorded GPS locations. The result will be a complete overview of how the user of the phone has been located relative to geographical units and their POIs, thus providing the necessary contextual information needed for data aggregation across a population of app users.

7.5.3 Local data aggregation on the phone

Once the locations are provided by the means described above, the compiled information can be communicated back to the server for the population-wide data aggregation. The most important efficiency gain has been perfectly parallel data processing, which will scale well as the numbers of users grow, provided sufficient capacity for data communication on the server side. However, one can do more locally, on the phone. To preserve privacy as much as possible and to present the aggregated data at spatial and temporal levels that match operative needs, the first steps of data aggregation can be conducted locally, on the phone. For instance, when the data processing identifies that the user of the phone was present at the Sanatoriet bus stop from 10:27 to 10:34, the data can be aggregated to coarser levels in time and space. For instance, the event could be recorded as a stay at any bus stop in BSU 4416, Akebakkeskogen, or even coarser, in the city quarter Nordre Aker. Instead of producing the exact timing of the event, the event could be denoted as a stay between 10:00 and 12:00 with a duration of less than 15 minutes. When this aggregation is carried out locally, on the phone, the finer details of the user's stay and movements that would be discarded anyway in the aggregation process do not need to leave the phone, thus reducing the privacy risk. Once these locally aggregated data arrive at the server and are combined with similar data from other app users, techniques such as k-anonymity and ε-DP can be applied to further strengthen the privacy of individuals.

For the most advanced types of aggregated data listed in Section 7.2, one needs to include the interaction between users who have been close enough for long enough to qualify as close contacts. As explained in Chapters 5 and 6, the presence of a close contact is stored by the Smittestopp app as Bluetooth events where two or more phones have been in direct contact. Since these events are timestamped and the length of each event can be computed, this information can be correlated with the GPS events in order to tag the Bluetooth event with the appropriate location data. Once this is done, the same procedures as described above should be able to associate a close contact with a geographical location, or, in particular, with a POI. One thing to bear in mind, though, is that close contacts can be one to many, and not only one to one. It is noted that the techniques for local data aggregation described above can also be applied to this type of data prior to communication with the server. Typically, this would result in the coarse-grained message 'a 15-minute or shorter contact between two people happened at a bus stop in "Nordre Aker" between 10:00 and 12:00'.

7.5.4 Improved privacy

The above statement about improved privacy assumes that there is no need for the actual GPS coordinates on the server side for other types of analyses. As documented in a recently published report [3], a modified version of Smittestopp can effectively support contact tracing based on Bluetooth data alone, without any GPS information. Therefore, the outlined approach to distributed data aggregation could be integrated with this revised version of Smittestopp not only to reduce computing times and improve scalability, but also to achieve a higher level of privacy. The outlined approach could also be combined with contact tracing based on Google/Apple Exposure Notifications (GAEN), although then as two separate apps, since GAEN prevents the integrated use of the GPS interface, even when restricted to local processing on the phone. It should also be noted that the distributed data aggregation outlined above can be extended to further reduce the privacy risk by introducing privacy-preserving algorithms on the phone, prior to sending information to the server. In particular, one could implement a differential privacy scheme on the phone, which would be an effective remedy for the privacy concern expressed by the committee that evaluated the initial Smittestopp design [4]. As discussed in Section 7.2.1, this would to some extent distort the information sent back to the server, possibly reducing the correctness of the population-wide aggregated data. Thus, one would need to tune the parameters of the algorithm such that one introduces enough uncertainty to shield the individual user, but not so much that it jeopardizes the quality of the aggregated data, for instance, with respect to making informed decisions on future pandemic interventions.

Increased transparency and user interaction. Another possibility would be to alert the user whenever a new batch of locally aggregated data is ready for transfer back to the server, and allow the user to review and possibly remove sensitive events from the aggregated data set before it is dispatched. The possibility of such user intervention would provide a very high level of transparency, and hopefully strengthen the trust in the app. The data review process could be the user's choice, meaning that the user can at any time opt to (a) trust the system and not review the data, (b) be asked to review the data within a reasonable time window before automatic dispatch, or (c) never send data before the users provides explicit confirmation.

Potential caveats. The distributed data aggregation outlined in this section has not been implemented, and therefore non-evident problems could arise in practical use. However, the two main obstacles for this scheme to work are (a) the processing power and battery capacity offered by the phone and (b) ensuring that the locally aggregated data are sent to the server in time for further aggregation into the population-wide data sets.

It is well known that Norway is a country with quick and wide uptake of new technology, especially with respect to telecommunications. Therefore, a large fraction of the population has access to relatively new and powerful mobile phones that are frequently used to stream music and video or to play games. Since these applications require a certain computational power, it is reasonable to assume that most phones could perform the necessary computations well. However, experimentation with a wide range of phone models and versions of their operating systems would be necessary to know this for sure.

When it comes to communication of the data back to the server in time for further compilation, this situation is similar to what was already present with the original

Smittestopp app's communication of GPS data to the server. In fact, it would be an improvement in terms of volume, since the aggregated data would be significantly smaller than the raw, unpruned data. However, the timing of communications would be crucial to ensure the availability of each phone's contributions at the server when the global aggregation of the current period takes place. This is a side effect of security concerns, meaning that aggregation cannot be redone later. To reduce the timing risk, one can tune the length of the time interval between each aggregation/-communication step. The amount of lost data would thus probably be reduced.

7.6 Conclusions and lessons learned

In this chapter, we presented the types of data that the Smittestopp system was expected to aggregate at the population level to meet the government's needs for planning and assessing pandemic interventions. This aggregation included the estimation of population dynamics over time for different categories of spatial locations, such as the density of people at shopping malls and bus stops during different periods of the day. Moreover, we described the aggregation procedures that were implemented before the project was halted, as well as the more advanced techniques that were planned for subsequent inclusion. In sum, these procedures would have provided a high level of privacy protection, based on binning spatial and temporal information to coarse levels and combinations of k-anonymity and ε-DP privacy.

Due to the volume of incoming raw data, the data aggregation would be a computationally demanding task. Observing positive experiences from testing both a Bluetooth-only version of Smittestopp and a prototype app based on the GAEN framework, it is now clear that future implementations of a contact tracing app can avoid the centralized storage of GPS events. In this context, we have proposed a distributed approach to data aggregation where each phone would locally aggregate information to coarse spatial and temporal levels before sending it to the server for population-wide aggregation. This approach mean that GPS events would not leave the phone. One would thus achieve improved computational scalability and one could further protect individuals' privacy by imposing random noise through ε-DP privacy locally, on the phone, prior to communication with the server. In addition, one could offer user-driven audits of the information before it was dispatched.

It should be noted that, in the original situation, before June 2020, this distributed aggregation would not have been meaningful, since the centralized storage of GPS events was seen as necessary to meet Smittestopp's specifications. At that time, the Google/Apple framework was not yet available or proven, and it was unclear whether approaches not built on that framework would need GPS information to help fix the inherent problem of sleeping iPhones not detecting contacts. In the first phase of the project, the exact specification of aggregated data sets to target had not yet converged, which also called for centralized processing. With the proven performance of Bluetooth-only contact tracing, for iPhones as well, the scenario has significantly changed in favour of distributed data aggregation locally, on the phones.

References

[1] C. Dwork, F. McSherry, K. Nissim, and A. Smith. Calibrating noise to sensitivity in private data analysis. In S. Halevi and T. Rabin, editors, *Theory of Cryptography*, pages 265–284, Berlin, Heidelberg, 2006. Springer Berlin Heidelberg.

[2] B. C. M. Fung, K. Wang, R. Chen, and P. S. Yu. Privacy-preserving data publishing: A survey of recent developments. *ACM Comput. Surv.*, 42:1–53, 2010.

[3] S. R. Laboratory and S. Metropolitan. Sammenligning av alternative løsninger for digital smittesporing (in Norwegian). Technical report, 2020.

[4] J. Lilleng, O. R. Lykkebø, B. Borud, Øyvind Indrebø, E. A. Arvesen, A. Slater, and E. S. Heimark. Endelig rapport for kildekodegjennomgang av løsning for digital smittesporing av koronaviruset (in Norwegian). Technical report, Helse- og omsorgsdepartementet, 2020.

[5] A. Machanavajjhala, J. Gehrke, D. Kifer, and M. Venkitasubramaniam. L-diversity: Privacy beyond k-anonymity. In *22nd International Conference on Data Engineering (ICDE'06)*, 2006.

[6] M. of Health and C. Services. Forskrift om digital smittesporing og epidemikontroll i anledning utbrudd av covid-19 (in Norwegian). https://www.regjeringen.no/contentassets/ 116076d9a39b473a97d97474048e1fb0/kgl.-res.-27.-mars- digital-smittesporing.pdf. (Accessed 2020-09-28).

[7] I. of publich health. Coronavirus modelling at the niph. https://www. fhi.no/en/id/infectious-diseases/coronavirus/coronavirus- modelling-at-the-niph-fhi/. (Accessed 2020-10-26).

[8] P. Samarati and L. Sweeney. Protecting privacy when disclosing information: k-anonymity and its enforcement through generalization and suppression. Technical report, 1998.

[9] J. Tang, A. Korolova, X. Bai, X. Wang, and X. Wang. Privacy loss in Apple's implementation of differential privacy on MacOS 10.12. *CoRR*, abs/1709.02753, 2017.

Printed in the United States
by Baker & Taylor Publisher Services